D1524404

Healthy Eating & Clean Food Recipes for Weight Loss & Health

Included are: Alkaline Mediterranean Cookbook, Paleo Salads & Alkaline Diet Recipes

By Elena Garcia

www.YourWellnessBooks.com

Disclaimer
A physician has not written the information in this book. It is advisable that you visit a qualified dietician so that you can obtain a highly personalized treatment for your case, especially if you want to lose weight effectively. This book is for informational and educational purposes only and is not intended for medical purposes. Please consult your physician before making any drastic changes to your diet.

All information in this book has been carefully researched and checked for factual accuracy. However, the author and publishers make no warranty, expressed or implied, that the information contained herein is appropriate for every individual, situation or purpose, and assume no responsibility for errors or omission. The reader assumes the risk, and full responsibility for all actions and the author will not be held liable for any loss or damage, whether consequential, incidental, and special or otherwise, that may result from the information presented in this publication.

The book is not intended to provide medical advice or to take the place of medical advice and treatment from your personal physician. Readers are advised to consult their own doctors or other qualified health professionals regarding the treatment of medical conditions. The author shall not be held liable or responsible for any misunderstanding or misuse of the information contained in this book. The information is not intended to diagnose, treat, or cure any disease.

If you suffer from any medical condition, are pregnant, lactating, or on medication, be sure to talk to your doctor before making any drastic changes in your diet and lifestyle.

Contents

BOOK 1 Alkaline Mediterranean Cookbook

47 Delicious Clean Food Recipes to Help You Enjoy a Healthy Lifestyle and Lose Weight without Feeling Deprived

By Elena Garcia

www.YourWellnessBooks.com

Healthy Eating Made Exciting, Tasty and Fun!

Welcome to the World of Alkaline-Mediterranean Eating. A simple, hybrid diet approach aimed at enriching your diet with delicious and nutritious foods.

So that you can easily:
-Enjoy a healthy lifestyle without feeling deprived
-Make healthy eating exciting and fun and enjoy delicious, nourishing meals with your family and friends (no more "dieting"!)
-Combine nutrient-packed alkaline vegetables and greens with quality animal products, to create optimal balance (and never feel bored again!)
-Start losing weight naturally, simply by improving the quality of your calories and consuming delicious foods that can speed up your metabolism (without going hungry or feeling like you have to give up your favorite foods forever, and without the "yo-yo" effect
-Enjoy more variety in your diet and never again torture yourself with some fad or starvation diets
-Become an excellent, healthy cook and have everyone love you for it
-Enjoy more energy naturally, by giving your body exactly what it needs to thrive
-Feel confident and empowered knowing that you eat your way to vibrant health, while, potentially, reducing the risk of many preventable diseases, simply by eating more nutritious and delicious foods
-Gain more focus – so that you can perform better at work and feel amazing in your body

My goal is to make it as simple and doable as possible. So, we will be diving right into it! You can expect a simple-to-follow recipe and healthy eating guide!

Here's exactly what you will learn from this little book, as I guide you step-by-step on your journey to wellness through balanced eating:

Alkaline diet and foods deciphered – in this section, we will quickly have a look at the alkaline diet and foods. This section alone has the power to radically improve your health! You see, no matter what your nutritional preferences are, you can always enrich your diet with more alkaline foods like healthy vegetables and greens (even if you're not a vegetarian).

Mediterranean diet and foods made simple –then, I will guide you through one of the most delicious and healthy diets ever created – the Mediterranean diet. I will also show you a few simple tweaks you can make to your diet today to start enjoying the Mediterranean diet lifestyle!

Finally, I will show you how you can combine the alkaline and Mediterranean diets so that you can create your own version of this hybrid diet.

The good news is that this new approach is very flexible. So, you don't need to stress out about complicated diets. You will quickly discover a few, easy-to-implement, flexible eating ideas based on the Alkaline and Mediterranean lifestyles.

For example – how to combine healing greens and vegetables with healthy protein and other superfood ingredients by creating mouth-watering dishes you will never get bored with! We are talking traditional Spanish dishes, such as paella, in a very healthy alkaline version, or delicious Greek-style salads you can make in 20 minutes or less (the more you practice, the quicker it gets).

***

Before we will get into the *Alkaline Mediterranean* hybrid diet, I would like to offer you free access to our *Wellness Lifestyle newsletter*.

When you sign up, you will receive free instant access to our book *Alkaline Paleo Superfoods for Optimal Nutrition*.
With *Alkaline Paleo Superfoods*, you will discover the best clean food combinations to help you create nutritious meals on a busy schedule.

You will also be receiving other valuable tips and recipes from me to help you stay on track so that you can create a healthy lifestyle you love.
You can sign up on the next page and become a successful reader at no cost!

Wellness Newsletter & Bonus eBook

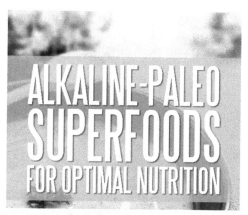

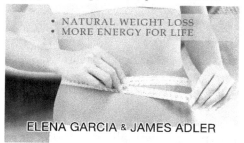

Sign up link:

www.yourwellnessbooks.com/newsletter

Problems with your download?
Contact us: elenajamesbooks@gmail.com

What the Heck Is This Alkaline Thing All About?

"Going green" is the way to describe an alkaline diet and lifestyle because the focus is on green vegetables in general, as they are the most alkaline foods you can possibly ingest.

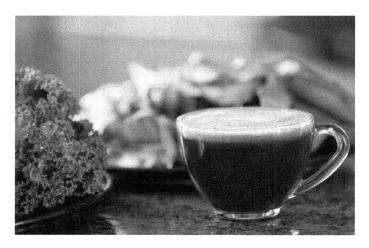

However, it's not about eating 100% green. That wouldn't be very doable!

It's all about adding more green, alkaline foods to your diet. This can be easily achieved by enriching your smoothies with leafy greens or adding a delicious salad to your meals. You can also add some leafy greens to your healthy (preferably made of low sugar ingredients) juices.

I have a couple of books dedicated to juices and smoothies (*Alkaline Ketogenic Juicing* & *Alkaline Ketogenic Smoothies*), in case you want to dive deeper into all kinds of healthy, healing concoctions.

This book, will also show you different ways to help you add more green, alkaline superfoods to your meals and drinks – almost on an autopilot!
There are multiple benefits of eating more alkaline:

Weight Loss
A diet rich in alkaline foods can assist you in losing weight. One way that it does this is obvious. The foods you will be eating are very healthy, rich in minerals, and low calorie in general.

Another benefit of an alkaline lifestyle regarding weight loss is that alkaline systems have more oxygen in their cells. Oxygen is a very essential part of eliminating fat cells from the body.

The more oxygen in your system, the more efficient your metabolism will be.

Natural Energy
Adding more greens into your diet does not only give you energy for the apparent reason that you are eating many more healthy, energizing vitamins. You are negating the acid-induced lethargy that is brought on by an unhealthy acid-forming diet (fast foods, sugar, processed carbohydrates etc.)

Not only do our bodies need an abundance of oxygen to lose weight, but we also need oxygen in our cells to energize us. The lack of oxygen in our cells causes fatigue. No, it is not just because you worked too late or partied to hard the night before. It is internal. If your cells are trying to function in a highly acidic environment, they will not be able to transfer oxygen efficiently; leading of course to exhaustion.

Cells in the body also make something that is called adenosine triphosphate (ATP). If your system is very acidic, it harms the ability of your cells to produce it. In the scientific world, it is known as the "energy currency of life." The ATP molecule contains the energy that we need to accomplish most things that we do (both internally and externally).

BODILY FUNCTIONS
Another benefit of the alkaline lifestyle is that your body will be able to function at an optimum level instead of being inhibited by acids:
-Your heartbeat is thrown off by acidic wastes in the body. The stomach suffers greatly from over-acidity.
-The liver's job is to get rid of acid toxins, but also to produce alkaline enzymes. By simply reducing your acid intake, you can internally boost your alkalinity thanks to your liver!

-Your pancreas thrives on alkalinity. Too much acid in your system throws off your pancreas. If you eat alkaline foods, your pancreas can regulate your blood sugars.
-Your kidneys also help to keep your body alkaline. When they are overwhelmed by an acidic diet, they cannot do their job
-The lymph fluids function most efficiently in an alkaline system. They remove acid waste. Acidic systems not only have a slower lymph flow causing acids to be stored; they can also cause acids to be reabsorbed through lymphatic ducts in your intestines that would typically be excreted.

MENTAL FOCUS
The alkalinity of the system is one of the best ways to focus and strengthen the mind. Just as the rest of the body is poorly affected by acid-forming foods and other toxins, so is your brain.

And as we all know, it should be possible to control your emotions and decision making with your mind. Guess what? If your body is too acidic and is not alkaline, your mental clarity will be cloudy, your decision making could be off, as well as your emotional state.

DETOX
Another huge benefit of an alkaline lifestyle is detoxification. First, you are going to be cutting out processed foods that are continually adding toxins to your system.

Secondly, you are going to be eating foods that allow your body to detox and rid itself of the acids that have built up in your system all this time. When we detoxify our bodies, our emotions, bodily functions, and mental functions can operate at their optimum levels.

Our bodies function optimally when our blood is at about 7.365 - 7.45 pH.

pH levels range from 0 to 14. 0 is the highest level of acidity, but basically, everything 0-7 would be considered acidic. The 7-14 range is alkaline.

Before we dive into complicated pH discussions, here is one thing to understand:

-The alkaline <u>diet is not about changing or "raising" your pH</u>. This is where many alkaline guides go wrong. You see, our body is smart enough to **self-regulate** our pH for us, no matter what we eat.

Unfortunately, when you constantly bombard your body with acid-forming foods (for example, processed foods, fast food, alcohol, sugar, and even too much meat), you torture your body with incredible stress. Why? Well, because it has to work harder to maintain that optimal pH...

Here's a simple example...

Imagine you immerse yourself in a bath filled with ice. You say, but hey, my body can self-regulate its optimal temperature, right? And yes, it can. But it will eventually collapse, and you will get ill. The same happens with nutrition and our blood pH.

You can spend years indulging in toxic, processed, acid-forming foods that only deprive your body of its vital nutrients, saying: "But hey, my body will self-regulate its optimal blood pH."

And again, it will...but sooner or later, it will give up and manifest a disease. It will accumulate fat as its natural defense function to protect your body from over-acidity. We don't wanna end up there, right?

Changing your diet to one that is full of alkaline foods is one of the easiest and best things you can do for your overall health. One of the easiest and most effective ways to do so is with salads. The good news is that you can say goodbye to boring, unappetizing, strictly alkaline salads make of broccoli, tomatoes, and cucumber.

We will be eating delicious and filling alkaline Mediterranean meals to get you closer to your health goals starting today!

Now, let's have a look at our alkaline food lists, so that you have a practical understanding of what alkaline foods and drinks look like. I also recommend you go to our private website at:

www.YourWellnessBooks.com/charts

and grab your printable alkaline food charts to stick on your fridge or keep in your car, to have it ready when you go shopping.

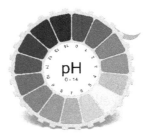

The recipes contained in this book are super rich in alkaline foods while taking advantage of traditional, Mediterranean clean-food recipes to help you create optimal balance and enjoy what you eat. If you don't enjoy it, it's hard to stick to it. That's my personal philosophy. Balance is key!

Ok, so now, let's have a look at our alkaline food lists:

Alkaline Veggies:

Asparagus
Broccoli
Chilli
Capsicum/Pepper
Courgette/Zucchini
Dandelion
Cabbage
Sweet Potato
Mint
Ginger
Coriander
Basil
Brussels Sprouts
Pumpkin
Radish
Snowpeas
Green Beans
String Beans
Runner Beans
Spinach
Kale
Cauliflower

Carrot
Beetroot
Eggplant/Aubergine
Garlic
Onion
Parsley
Butternut etc.)
Pumpkin
Wakame
Kelp
Collards
Chives
Endive
Chard
Celery
Cucumber
Watercress
Lettuce
Peas
Broad Beans
New Potato

ALKALINE SPROUTS:
Soy Sprouts
Alfalfa Sprouts
Amaranth Sprouts
Broccoli Sprouts
Fenugreek Sprouts
Kamut Sprouts
Mung Bean Sprouts
Quinoa Sprouts
Radish Sprouts
Spelt Sprout

ALKALINE FRUITS:
Avocado
Tomato
Lemon
Lime
Grapefruit
Fresh Coconut
Pomegranate

ALKALINE GRASSES:
Wheatgrass
Barley Grass
Kamut Grass
Dog Grass
Shave Grass
Oat Grass

ALKALINE NUTS AND SEEDS:
Almonds
Coconut
Flax Seeds
Pumpkin Seeds
Sesame Seeds
Sunflower Seeds

ALKALINE OILS:
Avocado Oil
Coconut Oil
Flax Oil
Udo's Oil
Olive Oil

ALKALINE BREAD:
Sprouted Bread
Sprouted Wraps
Gluten/Yeast
Free Breads & Wraps

ALKALINE BEANS AND GRAINS
Amaranth
Buckwheat
Chia/Salba
Kamut
Millet
Quinoa
Lentils
Mung Beans
Pinto Beans
Red Beans
Soy Beans
White Beans

Go to:

www.YourWellnessBooks.com/charts

to download your printable PDF alkaline charts to help you enrich your diet with alkaline foods!

Does Going Alkaline Mean I Have to Eat ONLY 100% Alkaline Foods, All the Time?

No, luckily, it's much easier (and more flexible) than that. When it comes to the alkaline diet, there is something called the 70/30 rule meaning that about 70% of your diet should be fresh, nutrient-dense alkaline-forming foods and the remaining 30% can be acid-forming foods (however they still should be clean and organic, for example, grass-fed meat or organic eggs).

This is what we will be doing in this book! We will be creating, Alkaline-Mediterranean hybrid diet...So that we can combine greens and other alkaline foods with quality non-alkaline foods (such as seafood, fish or meat).

Imagine, some fresh salmon, served with a large avocado, lime juice, and spices.

Or...an amazing veggie salad with some tuna and organic cheese.

It's all about balance!

The reason I have been able to live an alkaline lifestyle for so many years now, is because I follow the 70/30 rule (sometimes 80/20). I love combining alkaline diet and foods with other healthy diets (paleo, keto or, in our case – Mediterranean diet).

That being said, once a year, I like to go on an alkaline cleanse and then, I detox my body by eating super alkaline foods! It helps me heal my body, get rid of stubborn fat and feel more focus and energy.

To learn more about my favorite alkaline cleanse, visit:

www.YourWellnessBooks.com/cleanse

I truly believe it can help you on your journey to vibrant health (and sustainable weight loss, if that is your goal)

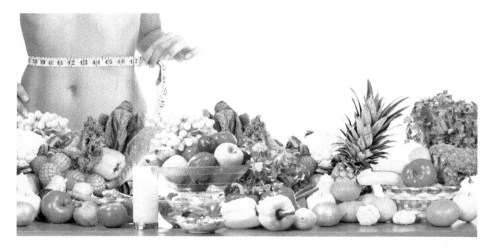

Now, let's have a look at the Mediterranean diet...

The Oldest and Most Proven Clean Food Approach Ever Created – the Mediterranean Diet

According to U.S. News & World Report the Mediterranean Diet is the best overall and easiest to follow.

It's still growing in popularity, with the latest research documenting its numerous benefits, and chefs and healthy food enthusiasts embracing Mediterranean ingredients and flavors.

It's basic run-down is this:

-Consume natural, organic, unprocessed foods
-Add more fruits and vegetables to your diet – serve your meals with fresh salads, and instead of snacking on processed sweets, snack on some fruit!
-Reduce the consumption of red meat to once a week. Add fish, seafood, and occasional white meat.
-Add good fats to your diet -avocadoes, organic olive oil, and avocado oil are very good for you.
-Reduce the consumption of sweets only for special occasions
-Choose organic, brown bread instead of a processed/ white.
-You can include quality dairy products in small amounts. Personally,

I like adding some quality goat cheese to my salads!

Add some nuts and seeds to your diet.

Legumes and lentils can also be turned into amazing Mediterranean dishes, as well! It's all about variety.

Make sure you drink enough water to stay hydrated, you can also make delicious smoothies (check out the recipes in the bonus section at the end of this book).

The Mediterranean Diet Benefits:
• Can prevent Parkinson's disease and Alzheimer's disease
• Reduces inflammation (it has an alkalizing effect on the body)

- Can prevent developing heart diseases
- Reduces risk of having stroke
- Improves mental and physical health and can even prevent depression and anxiety
- Is the best anti-ageing diet!

Combining Alkaline with Mediterranean
The basic rule to shift your meals towards an alkaline-Mediterranean friendly style is to:

-add more greens to your diet (can be done through salads, or you can juice the greens, or add them to your smoothies).

-add more good fats (for example fish, avocado, coconut oil)

Now, let's have a break from the theory and have a look at some delicious recipes to help you get started!

Recipe Measurements

I love keeping ingredient measurements as simple as possible- this is why I usually stick to tablespoons, teaspoons and cups.

The cup measurement I use is the American cup measurement. I also use it for dry ingredients. If you are new to it, let me help you:

If you don't have American Cup measures, just use a metric or imperial liquid measuring jug and fill your jug with your ingredient to the corresponding level. Here's how to go about it:
1 American Cup (1 c.)= 250ml= 8 fl.oz

For example:
If a recipe calls for 1 cup (1c.) of almonds, simply place your almonds into your measuring jug until it reaches the 250 ml/8oz mark.
I know that different countries use different measurements and I wanted to make things simple for you.

PART I

Vegetarian and Plant-Based Recipes

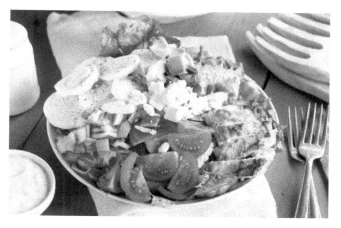

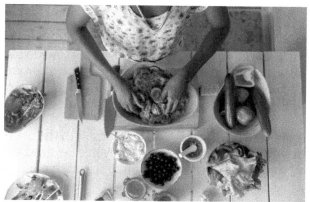

Easy Vegetable Frittata Recipe

This recipe is super quick to prepare. It makes a healthy and nutritious veggie meal! It is also super tasty and great for digestion. This recipe can be served as a quick and nutritious dinner.

Serves: 2-3
Ingredients:
- 5 tbsp. olive oil (extra virgin)
- Total veggies=2 cups (use any amount of each: spinach, asparagus, kale, broccoli, mushrooms etc.)
- 1/2 red onion, diced
- 1 tbsp. parsley, chopped
- 2 garlic cloves, minced
- 6 large organic eggs
- 1/8 c. grated parmesan
- ½ tsp. black pepper
- Pinch of salt

Instructions:
1. Set your oven to 400 Fahrenheit (or 200 Celsius)
2. Using a pan that you can put in the oven, heat (over medium) the 1 tbsp. of olive oil and add the garlic and onion, brown for about three minutes. Now put in all of the other vegetables. Cook for 4-6 min depending on how you like them. Salt and pepper them.
3. In a separate bowl, whisk up the eggs with the cheese and pour them onto the veggies, so that they are covered evenly.
4. Now, put into the oven and bake for about ten min or until eggs are done. Enjoy!

Nutritious Eggs n' Asparagus

Asparagus and garlic have an alkalizing effect on this meal which makes it a perfectly balanced and healthy combination. The Alkaline-Mediterranean diet loves combining alkaline plant-based foods with quality animal products to create a perfect balance!

This recipe can be served as a quick breakfast, brunch or lunch.

Serves: 2-3
Ingredients:
- 6 organic eggs
- 30 trimmed asparagus, halved
- 1 1/2 cup sauce (recipe below)
- 1 tbsp. organic olive oil
- 1 clove garlic, minced
- 2 cups vegetable broth
- 1/4 cup Pecorino Romano, grated

Instructions:
1. Heat a large skillet to medium.
2. Add the olive oil and sauté your garlic. Let it brown, only cook for 2-3 minutes.
3. Stir in the sauce and broth with the garlic and blend them well.
4. Throw in your asparagus pieces, cover with a lid.
5. When the sauce begins to simmer, add the cheese and eggs.
6. Turn to low and simmer for ten minutes.
7. Enjoy!

Sauce:
- 2 cups canned plum tomatoes, drain, seed and cut into quarter inch strips
- 3 tbsp. evoo (extra virgin olive oil) 1 heaping tbsp. basil
- 1 tsp minced garlic cloves
- 1/8 tsp. salt
- 1/8 tsp. crushed red pepper

Sauce instructions:
Put everything into a medium sized skillet and heat to medium-high. Simmer for five min. or until most of the liquid is gone.

Toast to the Greek Breakfast or Snack

This is a delicious, healthy dessert or snack that takes only 5 minutes to prepare. I also like it for breakfast or after workouts.
It's tasty, naturally sweet and rich in protein.

Serves: 1
Ingredients:
- 2 Tablespoons of organic Greek yogurt, no added sugar
- 1 piece of organic toast (bread recipe below)
- 1 Tablespoon of raw honey
- 1 Tablespoon of pistachios (no shell)

Instructions:
1. Use the Greek yogurt as a spread.
2. Top with the honey and some pistachios!
3. Enjoy!

Greek Loaf Organic Bread Recipe

Nothing feels better than preparing your own bread. This process can be time-consuming so make sure you schedule it on your day off, or when you have more free time.

Ingredients:

- 1 ounce of fresh yeast or (2 tbsp. dry)
- 1/2 cup warm water
- Whole wheat flour (separate from the amount to follow) ½ cup
- 8 cups whole wheat flour
- 1 tbsp. salt
- 2.5 cup warm water
- 2 tbsp. milk
- 2 tbsp. olive oil (extra virgin)
- 1 ½ - 2 tbsp. raw honey

Instructions:

1. Dissolve your yeast in a bowl with the ½ c. warm water.
2. Add the half cup flour; do it slowly while mixing well.
3. Mix until it is not lumpy and is thick in consistency.
4. Set aside and allow it to rise for 15-20 min.
5. In a big mixing bowl, sift the other flour and salt, make a crater in the middle.
6. Put the honey, oil and yeast flour, and 2 cups water into it.
7. Slowly, pull the flour into the moist middle with your hands until it is well mixed, add more of the last half cup water if needed a little bit at a time.
8. Flour a working area and knead the dough until it does not stick to your hands.
9. Put your dough in a bowl that is lightly greased and roll it in the oil.
10. Cover your bowl with a dry towel, then a damp towel, and another dry towel over that one. Allow to sit and double in size for two hours.
11. Take out and place on a floured work area. Punch it and then knead the dough for five min. or so. Divide into three or four loaves. Shape into loaf of your liking and put onto ungreased baking sheets. Cover with 3 dishtowels as before and let them rise again for one hour.

12. Heat your oven to 425 Fahrenheit (or: 210 Celsius)
13. If you like, you can score the tops of the loaves 3 times for a crustier loaf. Place them right on the rack in the center of the oven for 35 minutes, or less if looking too browned. It should sound hollow if you tap it on the bottom.
14. Cool on racks and enjoy!
15. You can use it for sandwiches, toast, and bruschetta as well!

From Regular Yogurt to Greek Yogurt:

You can use yogurt tied up in cheesecloth setting in a draining bowl, or buy a yogurt strainer.

1. Line a mixing bowl with cheesecloth.
2. Put your yogurt into the middle.
3. Pull up the sides of the cloth and twist it so that the yogurt is completely encased.
4. Twist the top corners of the cloth in order to strain out the liquid over the sink. Do this until you get most of the moisture out.
5. When it begins to barely drip, tie it up tight.
6. Set in a colander over a bowl in your refrigerator for a few hours or overnight.
7. Place in the sink and press out any leftover moisture.
8. Open it up and scoop into a bowl. It should be thick like sour cream.
9. It also tastes great with nuts and berries! Find your favorite combinations!

Vitamize Yourself Up Mediterranean Fruit Salad

A natural fruit salad is a much better and healthier alternative to eating processed sweets and cakes.

It's easy to make and naturally energizing! I love it for breakfast or as a quick afternoon snack with some nut milk, or nut butter.

Serves: 2-3

Ingredients:
- One pint of strawberries
- A papaya
- ½ of a pineapple
- An orange
- A whole custard apple
- A mango
- A lemon
- 2 Tablespoons of raw honey

Instructions:
1. First, peel the mango, pineapple, and papaya. Chop them all up into one-inch pieces.
2. Put them in a large bowl.
3. Rinse your strawberries and take off the tops. Cut each into fours, then throw them in the bowl.
4. Squeeze both the orange and the lemon juice over the fruit, then add the honey and stir to blend all ingredients. Refrigerate for an hour or more.

Here is another version of this recipe, where you can add different fruits, just keep the quantities the same.

Ingredients:
- 2 cup pineapple chopped into one in. pieces
- 2 cup mango chopped into one in. pieces
- 2 cup papaya cut into strips
- 2 cup kiwi quarter and cut into half inch pieces
- 25 cherries, pitted and halved
- 2 cup peaches chopped into one in. pieces
- 1 cup peeled oranges seeded and sliced
- 1 cup peeled tangerines seeded and sliced
- 4 tbsp. fresh lime juice
- 4 tbsp. sugar
- 10 tbsp. water
- 1 pinch of salt
- 1 tbsp. lime zest

Instructions:
1. Mix up the water and sugar in a small pot and allow to come to a boil, make sure it dissolves. Stir and allow to thicken.
2. Take the pan off of the heat and stir in zest; allow to cool.
3. Mix all of the fruit up in a big bowl and lightly salt. Add the lime sugar syrup. Toss the salad just a bit.
4. Cover the bowl and refrigerate for about two hours.
5. Serve with slotted spoon and enjoy!

Energizing Lentils n' Rice

This is a great, comforting meal for cold winters! It can be served for dinner, or even as a quick brunch.

Quinoa is a recommended alkaline grain as it's naturally gluten-free, rich in many nutrients and an excellent source of natural protein.

Serves: 2-4
Ingredients:

- 1 cup quinoa
- 1 cup green lentils
- ½ tsp Himalayan salt
- 4 cup water or veggie broth
- 2 large carrots
- Tahini if you like
- 1 teaspoon Italian spices blend

Instructions:

1. Go through the lentils and remove anything else that is in there.
2. Rinse them well under cold water. Get out a large to medium pot, put in the lentils and set on the stove.
3. Now, rinse the quinoa and add with your salt and water/broth.
4. Chop up your carrots and throw them in too.
5. Turn the heat up to high until the pot boils and then turn it down to lower setting. Keep it simmering, covered, for 45 min.
6. Add in the spices.
7. Turn off the stove and allow it to sit. Enjoy!

Nutritious Butternut Squash Salad

This delicious and nutritious recipe makes an excellent dinner and is just perfect for long, winter evenings.

Serves: 2-3
Ingredients:
- 3/4 cup quinoa
- 3-4 carrots (3 if large)
- Half cup lentils
- Half cup raisins
- 1 butternut squash (large ones are best for this recipe)
- 3 tbsp. extra virgin olive oil
- 2 tbsp. tahini
- 1 lime
- Pinch of salt/pepper
- Splash of apple cider vinegar
- 1 tbsp. rosemary (dried)

Instructions:
1. Preheat oven to 375 Fahrenheit (or 190 Celsius)
2. Take your squash and peel it, then slice in up into 1 in. pieces.
3. Put it on a baking tray. Drizzle over oil, along with salt and pepper to your liking. Cook for thirty minutes.
4. Cook quinoa and lentils together with water and ACV. Approximately 15 minutes.
5. Soak the raisins in a bowl of warm water.
6. Grate your carrots after peeling them.
7. Mix up the tahini, juice from the lime, and olive oil with a fork in a separate bowl.
8. Put everything into a large bowl, put the dressing on top. Toss well and enjoy!

__Aromatic Avocado Toast__

This outside the box, vegan-friendly toast makes an excellent breakfast – it's easy, nutritious and smells fantastic! It can also be used as a take-away lunch or brunch.

Serves: 1
First Variation:
Ingredients:
- Hummus (use store bought or one of the recipes in this book)
- Pesto (recipe in book)
- ¼ of a sliced cucumber
- ¼ cup sprouts
- 1 avocado (peeled, sliced, and pitted)
- Two slices of whole grain or wheat bread (you can use the Greek bread recipe if you like)

Instructions:
1. Toast two bread slices.
2. Spread the toast with some hummus.
3. Top with some pesto.
4. Lay cucumber on top of the pesto, add the sprouts, and then lay avocado on the very top of everything else.
5. Enjoy!!!!

Second Variation:
- Hummus (olive recipe)
- 8 sliced cherry tomatoes
- Pesto
- 1 avocado peeled, pitted, sliced
- Handful of sliced up baby spinach
- 2 pieces of toast (whole wheat/whole grain)

1. Toast the bread.
2. Spread the hummus and top with pesto
3. Place on the avocado, tomato, then the spinach.
4. Enjoy!

Alkaline Vegan Mediterranean Bean Salad

Salad is a great way of accompanying all your meals to help you add in more nutrients so that you can look and feel amazing.

Serves:3
Ingredients:
- 1 can of cannellini beans, rinse and drain well
- 1 avocado, peel, pit and dice
- 1/2 cup yellow onion, dice
- 1 carrot, chop
- 1/2 cup spinach, slice thin
- ½ cup thinly sliced kale
- Splash of ACV (apple cider vinegar)
- Juice of one lemon
- 1 Tablespoon of fresh orange juice
- Pinch of orange zest
- 1 Tablespoon shelled hemp seeds
- ¼ teaspoon cayenne
- Salt/pepper to your liking
- A few Tablespoons fresh chives
- Some kind of toasted bread

Instructions:
1. In large bowl mash up beans and avocado with a fork.
2. When it is a nice creamy, chunky consistency it is ready.
3. Fold in all of the veggies.
4. Whisk up the juice and vinegar and fold this into the vegetable to combine well.
5. Allow to chill for one half hour.
6. Enjoy atop your toast!

Home-Made Pita Bread

Enough to make 6 pitas. I like making them on Sundays to make sure I have fresh pita bread for my family for the whole week!

Ingredients:
- 2 cups water (warm)
- 4 tsp. instant yeast
- 1 tablespoon salt
- 4 cups flour (organic whole-wheat)

Instructions:
1. Mix water and yeast in a large bowl. Allow to set 5 minutes.
2. Slowly add salt and flour while stirring. Cover with a dishtowel and allow rising to occur for an hour.
3. Take out and put onto floured area. Knead it gently and re-cover for a half hour.
4. Set oven to 500 Fahrenheit (260 Celsius).
5. Split up the dough into 6 balls.
6. Roll out into eight-inch circles, as carefully as possible on one side.
7. Put the pita onto greased baking sheets and bake in the bottom half of your oven for 9 min. They should puff-up and be light brown.
8. You can cut them and open them or just use as bread! Enjoy!

Delicious Zucchini-Crust Veggie Pizza

This simple pizza recipe is yet another tasty way to help you add more veggies to your diet. Enjoy!

Serves:2
Ingredients:
- 4 cup fresh zucchini- grate and then chop - about 1 large or 3 very small zucchini
- 1/2 cup finely grated Mozzarella
- 5 tablespoons of almond meal
- 3 tablespoons fresh grated Parmesan
- 1 teaspoon oregano, dry Greek
- ½ teaspoon garlic powder
- ¼ teaspoon salt
- 1 egg, beat well
- 1/2 cup pesto sauce (recipe in book)
- 1-6 oz. jar artichokes, drain then chop
- 1/3 cup re-hydrated sun-dried tomatoes, slice
- ½ cup Kalamata olives, chop
- ½ cup spinach
- ¼ cup thin sliced red onion

Instructions:
1. Set oven to 450 Fahrenheit (or 240 Celsius).
2. Grate the zucchini with the large holes on a grater. Now chop it all up.
3. Put it in a bowl and put in the microwave for five minutes on high.
4. Line a strainer with a towel and allow it to drain until cool.
5. Squeeze the zucchini in the cloth to remove moisture. Then put it in a mixing bowl.
6. Mix in your cheeses, almond meal, garlic, oregano, salt and egg until well-combined.
7. Grease a cookie sheet with olive oil.
8. Divide crust in two and press it out by hand. Do not make it too thin.
9. Bake until it is firm and barely beginning to brown.
10. Turn oven down to 400 Fahrenheit (or 200 Celsius).
11. Top each crust with pesto and toppings and bake when oven is down to 400, just long enough for veggies to soften (5-10 min).

Hummus Extravaganza

Nothing tastes better than home-made hummus.
This recipe is enough to make about 2- 3 cups of deliciously fresh hummus. You can serve it with veggies (carrots, cucumbers), rice dishes, or on a piece of toast.

Makes: 2.5 Cups
Ingredients:
- Fresh juice from two lemons
- One half cup water (from the cooking of the beans)
- 6 tablespoons Tahini
- 2 tablespoons extra virgin olive oil
- Two cups cooked garbanzo beans, soaked overnight and simmered a few hours, remove skins (optional) (save the water)
- 2/3 cup Kalamata olives, take out the pits
- 2- 3 cloves of garlic, peel
- ½ teaspoon of salt
- Pinch of cayenne pepper

Instructions:
1. Mix the lemon with the water.
2. Using another bowl, whisk up the tahini and olive oil until they are smooth and well-blended.
3. Throw the garbanzos, cloves of garlic, olives and the cayenne pepper into your food processor or blender until they are smooth. Keep scraping the stuff off of the sides.
4. Keep the processor on and slowly add the lemon juice, mixed with the cooking water, for one min. Then keep scraping down the bowl.
5. Now do the same with the tahini and oil.
6. When it is smooth, put in a bowl and cover. Put in the fridge for an hour or so to let the flavors blend.
7. Enjoy with some home-made pitta bread (in moderation), or fresh veggies (in abundance!).

You can also eat this super delicious hummus on fresh veggies, sandwiches, wraps, salads, etc.

Easy Spicy Lentil Soup

Do you like spicy food? Try this amazing lentil soup. I recommend it for cold winter evenings. It has a nice, oriental touch that is energizing and refreshing!

Serves: 2-3
Ingredients:
- 3 tbsp. extra virgin olive oil
- 1 big red onion, chop
- 1 large carrot, chop
- 1 jalapeño, seed and chop up
- 1 1/4 cup lentils (brown) rinsed
- 2 leaves of bay
- 1 tsp oregano
- 2 tsp paprika
- 1/2 teaspoon ground cumin
- ¼ tsp of cayenne
- 1.5 cup tomatoes, diced (canned or fresh)
- 1 tbsp. tomato-paste
- 1 cup veggie broth
- 1 tsp salt
- 1 tsp fresh black pepper
- Chopped parsley (about a handful) red wine vinegar, and extra oil for serving.

Instructions:
1. Put the oil in a large pot and turn heat to medium. Put in the onion sauté for three minutes.
2. Next throw in the carrot and jalapeño. Cook, constantly stirring for three more minutes.
3. Put in your lentils, bay, spices, tomatoes/tomato paste, and the veggie broth. Turn up the heat and allow to boil, then turn to low. Put a lid on it. Allow it to simmer 45 minutes.
4. You may want to add more water.
5. Salt and pepper to your liking. Right before serving, add the parsley and a bit of the vinegar and oil.
6. Enjoy hot!

Aromatic Veggie Lasagne

This simple, and very aromatic veggie-style lasagne is designed to help you get hooked on veggies!

Serves: 4
Ingredients:
- 2 teaspoons olive oil
- 2 garlic cloves, mince
- 1 onion, dice
- 1 pound crimini mushrooms, slice
- 2-15 ounce cans of diced tomatoes (salt-free)
- ¼ teaspoon of salt
- 2 teaspoons of basil, dry
- 1 teaspoon of oregano, dry
- 1 teaspoon of thyme, dry
- Olive oil to grease
- 1.5 pound of eggplant, slice into thin circles
- 8 ounces of mozzarella sliced

Instructions:
1. Put the oil into a large frying pan and heat to medium-high.
2. Put the garlic in with the oil for two minutes, stirring the duration of that time.
3. Put in your onion, cooking another four min. Keep up the stirring.
4. Now put in the mushrooms and allow to cook for ten min.
5. Next, put in the salt, canned tomatoes, and herbs. Turn down the heat to medium. Put a lid on and simmer for about ten minutes. Make sure to stir a few times.
6. Uncover and stir for about 15 more min. Make sure you are stirring.
7. Set your oven to 325 Fahrenheit (or 160 Celsius).
8. Use a 9 x 13 pan and oil it.
9. Spread a layer, using half of the eggplant in the pan. Pour in half of your sauce.
10. Put in the rest of the eggplant as the next layer and then cover with the other half of the sauce.
11. Put foil on top and bake for a half of an hour.
12. Turn up the oven to 375 Fahrenheit (or 190 Celsius) and bake another half of an hour.

43

13. Take off the foil, lay cheese over the top and bake for ten more minutes.
14. Allow to set for 5 min and serve.

Catalan Dream Extravaganza

This is a great family dessert that everyone will enjoy! It's naturally dairy-free, but still very creamy and delicious.

Serves: 4
Ingredients:
- l cup almond milk or rice milk
- 6 medium eggs yolks
- 1 cup of brown, organic sugar
- 2 tablespoons of starch or cornstarch
- 1 cinnamon stick
- The skin of half a lemon

Instructions:
1. Wash and brush the lemon peel. Peel avoiding the white part because it has a bitter taste.
2. Dilute cornstarch or starch in your chosen milk (about half a cup)
3. Pour the remaining milk in a saucepan and boil with the cinnamon stick and lemon peel. Remove from heat, cover and infuse warm to leave.
4. Meanwhile, whisk the egg yolks with sugar until white and mix with milk.
5. Add the cup of milk diluted with starch, mix well and let it cook on low heat, while still stirring until thick and creamy.
6. Remove the cream from heat ,take away the lemon peel and cinnamon and pour the cream into a wide source or small molds.
7. Cool the cream and set aside in the mold.
8. Put in the fridge and serve cold.
9. Serve with cinnamon and raw almonds if you wish. I also like adding a few raisins.

Melanzane Mozarella Dream

This dish requires rather long prep time- up to 2 and a half hours so make sure that you have someone to lend you a hand! Enjoy a nice conversation when cooking or treat yourself to a glass of organic wine.

Serves:4
Ingredients:
- 4 medium eggplants
- Half a kilo of ripe tomatoes
- 1 cup of fresh mozzarella cheese (check out in Italian food store to get the best one)
- 2 garlic cloves
- 2 tbsp. grated Parmesan cheese
- 3 sprigs of basil
- 4 tbsp. of virgin olive oil
- pepper
- sea salt or Himalayan salt

Instructions:
1. Wash the eggplant and dry it with a clean cloth and remove the stems from the tops.
2. Cut the eggplant, don't peel it, and slice it very thin.
3. Arrange the slices in a colander and sprinkle with salt. Let them drain for an hour to release the bitter juice out. Then, rinse quickly under running water and dry them carefully.
4. Peel and chop the garlic and tomatoes.
5. Cut the mozzarella into thin slices
6. Heat 2 tablespoons oil in a skillet over low heat and sauté the garlic.
7. Add the chopped tomato and basil. Add salt and pepper and sauté over medium heat for 10 minutes.
8. Finish the sauce by passing it through the food mill and set aside.
9. Stir fry the eggplant in batches adding more olive oil if necessary. Set aside when it gets brownish.
10. Finally, prepare for baking:
11. Arrange a layer of eggplant in the bottom of your baking dish and cover with a few tablespoons of tomato sauce and parmesan cheese.

12. Top with a cover of mozzarella (sliced). Then cover with tomato sprinkled with parmesan and bake for about 30-40 minutes in a preheated oven at 360 Fahrenheit (or 180 Celsius).
13. You can serve it warm or cold.

Kale Minestrone

Who said that eating vegetables is boring? I can never get bored of this recipe. Feel free to experiment with your favorite spices to make this dish unique and to slightly transform it whenever you feel like!

Serves:4
Ingredients:
- 1 large red onion, chopped
- 3 carrots, diced
- 2 stalks of celery, diced
- 3-4 cloves of garlic, minced
- 3 potatoes, dice (1/2 in.) and rinsed
- 1 zucchini, sliced (half circles)
- 2 1/2 cups beans (cannellini), cooked or 2 cans, drain and rinse
- 1 can tomatoes, diced
- 1/2 cup quinoa or whole wheat pasta (uncooked)
- 2 cups kale, torn and tightly packed
- 7 cups boiling veggie broth
- 2 bay leaves
- 1 tablespoon oregano, dried
- ½ tablespoon dry thyme
- ½ tablespoon fresh rosemary
- ½ tsp cayenne pepper
- Salt/pepper to your liking

Instructions:
1. Get out a large soup pot and heat to medium high with two tablespoons of water in the bottom. The water will begin to boil, so you then need to put in onion, carrot, celery, and cloves of garlic. Allow them to cook for 7 minutes and stir often. You may need to put in extra water to keep veggies from sticking.
2. Boil the veggie broth in another pot and turn off heat.
3. In the first large soup pot, put in the potato, zucchini, tomatoes, bay, spices, and cannellini beans. Keep the temperature at medium high and keep stirring so that everything gets hot.
4. Put in the veggie stock. Put a lid on and let it boil. Then turn down and simmer for 15 min. (IF using quinoa add now)

5. If using pasta, add now along with the rosemary, allow to cook for five min.
6. Next, it is time to put in your kale along with salt and pepper to your liking. Stir and then allow the soup to sit, covered, for ten minutes before eating.
7. Enjoy!

Italian Classic Pesto

Pesto is delicious and naturally alkalizing. While it's traditionally eaten with pasta, you can also use it for your toasts, salads, quinoa, and veggies. You can also serve it with some spiralized carrots or zucchini. So yummy and healthy!

Ingredients:
- 2 cups fresh sweet basil leaves
- ½ cup extra virgin olive oil
- 3 tbsp. pine nuts
- Himalayan salt to taste
- Total amount of cheese needs to=¼ c. use Pecorino Romano and/or Parmigianino cheese.

Instructions:
1. Boil a pot of water with salt in it. While it is boiling, make a big ice bath in your sink.
2. When you see the water boiling, add your basil. Do this in several different batches. Leave each batch in the water for eight second and remove right away dunking straight into the ice water. Use a salad-spinner to drain or dry with paper towels.
3. Toast the nuts in a pan over medium heat until aromatic. Allow them to cool on a plate.
4. Crush your garlic cloves while the nuts cool and then blend all in the food processor.
5. Next put the blanched basil in with the pine nut and garlic blend. Process on high.
6. Slowly add the remaining oil and salt. Now add the cheese. Blend until it is a smooth as you like it to be.
7. Keep stored in containers in the fridge with a touch of olive oil.

Qui-zpacho

This is a combination of Spanish gazpacho and quinoa – the perfect recipe for a quick and nourishing meal.

Serves:4
Ingredients:
- ¾ of a bell pepper, de-seed
- ½ of a cucumber, peeled and sliced
- 2 ½ -3 cloves of garlic, chopped
- 1/4 cup of extra virgin olive oil
- 1 cup of cooked quinoa
- 6 tomatoes, peeled then quartered
- ½ tablespoon sea salt
- ½ tsp. red wine vinegar
- ¼ tsp. extra virgin olive oil

Instructions:
1. Put bell pepper in a blender. The garlic and cucumber are to be put in now as well. Only put 1/2 cup of the olive oil in there and blend until smooth.
2. Add quinoa, a little at a time, blending until smooth. Add tomato one at a time and keep blending until super smooth. Put into a bowl and add salt and cayenne. Cover and put in the fridge for 1 hour or more.
3. When serving, drizzle ¼ tsp. olive oil and some balsamic over each.

Alkaline-Mediterranean Basil-Tomato Bruschetta Topping

This is a simple, light dish that makes a perfect aperitif or a quick, refreshing, alkaline-rich snack.

People often ask me why tomatoes are considered alkaline-forming to the body. After all, aren't they acidic?

Well, yes, they taste acidic. However, they have an alkaline-forming effect on the body (it's because of the fact that they are very low in sugar and high in alkaline minerals, such as potassium). Exactly what your body needs to stay in optimal balance!

Ingredients:
- 1-1/2 lb. ripe tomatoes (about 5), cut into 1/4-inch pieces
- salt
- Pinch cayenne
- 1 clove garlic with a bit of oil mashed into a paste
- 2 leafy sprigs basil, chop roughly

Instructions:
1. Sprinkle salt over the tomatoes.
2. Drain them in a colander for ten minutes.
3. Put them in a bowl and lightly stir in the garlic, oil, and basil.
4. Sprinkle cayenne and fold in.
5. Enjoy! Goes well with a bottle of Sauvignon Blanc!

Whole Wheat Pita Pockets

Whole wheat, home-made pita pockets can be a great addition to your vegetable soups and creams. Use them as a special treat!

Makes 8 servings
Ingredients:
- 3 ½ cup whole wheat flour
- 1 tbsp. active dry yeast
- ¼ cup water (warm)

Instructions:
1. Set oven to 500 degrees Fahrenheit (or 260 Celsius) and allow to preheat.
2. In a bowl, sift 2 cups of your flour with the yeast.
3. Once the dry ingredients are combined, mix in the water.
4. Add the other 1 ½ cups of flour slowly until the dough comes loose from the sides of the mixing bowl.
5. Now it is time to knead your dough. Knead well for four minutes.
6. Take out your dough and make it into eight evenly sized balls.
7. Flour a counter top or a large cutting board. Use a rolling pin and make each ball into a five or six in. circle. Do not roll them thinner than ¼ inch.
8. Spread some flour on each side of the pita.
9. Put each one on a non-stick cookie sheet and let them rise for a half hour.
10. Flip each one over carefully. Be sure not to pinch the edge or jostle them around too much.
11. Put them in the oven on the bottom rack and cook for five minutes, then remove.

Easy Spanish Aioli

This creamy-style dip is delicious, nutritious and healthy. It's traditionally served with seafood, however you can also use it as a bread spread or serve it with some veggies.
It also tastes delicious with fried potatoes!

Ingredients:
- 7 cloves of garlic, chop
- 1/2 tsp. salt
- 1 tsp. freshly squeezed lemon juice
- 2 eggs (yolks only)
- 2/3 cup olive oil
- 1 tablespoon fresh oregano, chop

Instructions:
1. Put your oregano, salt and the garlic into the processor and mix well.
2. Put in the lemon juice and egg, pulse again.
3. Slowly drizzle the oil into the food processor and pulse well.

Almost Alkaline Greek Salad

This salad combines balance, nutrition and taste. It always feels good to combine the healing benefits of alkaline veggies with super tasty Mediterranean ingredients.

Serves:2
Ingredients:
- 1 pound chickpeas, soaked and cooked
- 5 tomatoes (big ones)
- 1 cucumber (large)
- 14 olives (Kalamata)
- 1 big red onion
- 1 bell pepper
- 1-4 oz. piece of feta cheese
- Some extra virgin olive oil
- Some dry oregano (Greek)
- Some red wine vinegar
- Pinch salt

Instructions:
1. Wedge tomatoes.
2. After peeling your cucumber, slice into half inch circles and half them.
3. Slice the onion up very thin.
4. Mix the tomato and cucumber together in a bowl. Add chickpeas and top with the onion and olives,
5. Now drizzle with oil and a bit of vinegar (2:1).
6. Add salt if you like.
7. Last step is to place a slice of feta on top and sprinkle the oregano.
8. Enjoy!

Greek Quinoa Salad

This is yet another delicious example of vegetarian-style alkaline-Mediterranean dishes. Quinoa is a miracle grain, it's super nutritious, rich in protein and a perfect ingredient for super healthy salads like this one. Pine nuts, mint and cheese give this salad an incredible taste!

Serves:3-4
Ingredients:
- 1 1/2 cups quinoa
- 6 cups of kale, chop
- 1 red pepper, chopped
- ¼ c. pine nuts
- 4 oz. sphela cheese, crumbled
- 1 lemon
- 1/4cup chopped mint
- 1 ½ cups red grapes, halved
- Extra virgin olive oil

Instructions:
1. To make the quinoa: Bring 1 1/2 cups of rinsed quinoa and three cups of water to a boil. Now turn to low, simmering covered for 15 minutes. Put the quinoa in a bowl in the refrigerator to cool.
2. In a bowl, marinate the kale with the lemon juice for a half hour.
3. Toss in all of the other ingredients (hold off on the oil).
4. When everything is well-tossed, you should drizzle the oil over the entire salad.
5. Enjoy!

Easy Italian Berry-Bean Salad

Berries are an excellent (but very often overlooked) salad ingredient and they taste delicious with some honey and balsamic vinegar.

Serves: 3-4
Ingredients:
- 1-16 oz. can green beans
- 1-16 oz. can chickpeas
- 1-16 oz. can kidney beans
- 1 whole bell pepper, slice
- 3 stalks of celery, chop
- 1 onion (green), chop
- 1 cup total berries of your choice, fresh or frozen
- 1/4 cup balsamic vinegar
- 3 tablespoons honey
- 1 lemon (juice from)
- 1 tbsp. extra virgin olive oil

Instructions:
1. Drain all of the beans and put into a big bowl. Mix in bell pepper, celery and the onion. Combine well.
2. In a blender or food processor blend berries, vinegar, honey, lemon, and olive oil.
3. Pour over the bean salad. Toss and allow to marinate for the night in the refrigerator.
4. Enjoy!

Italian Style Farro Salad

This recipe makes a very creative, nutritious and delicious dinner salad that is very likely to surprise all your guests!

Serves:4
Ingredients:
- 14 ounces farro
- 6 cups of vegetable stock
- 3 very ripe tomatoes, dice
- 12 leaves of basil (chopped)
- 4 garlic cloves, crush well
- 1/4 cup extra virgin olive oil (for cooking the vegetables, set aside 3 tbsp.)
- Salt and crushed red pepper to taste
- 1 large zucchini, slice
- 1 large red onion, dice
- 1 bell pepper, dice
- 1 eggplant (a smaller one)

Instructions:
1. Rinse the farro and remove anything bad in there.
2. Heat 3 tbsp. oil for cooking the veggies in the bottom of a pot to medium. Now add the garlic and farro. Sautee the garlic until it is golden brown, and toast the farro as well. Keep stirring so that it does not stick.
3. Now, add the veggie stock, a few spoonfuls at a time. Keep stirring while you are adding the broth, it will be evaporating. When farro is soft, it is done.
4. Heat up 4 tbsp. oil in another pan to medium. Mix the red onion, zucchini, pepper, eggplant, and tomato. Salt and sauté until they are soft. If you run out of moisture in the pan, add a tad of veggie stock.
5. When the vegetables are done, take them off the stove and mix them in with the farro.
6. Add basil and crushed red pepper. Plate and drizzle with oil if you like.
7. Enjoy! A glass of Rosé? Yes please!

Nutty Aromatic Romesco Dip/Sauce

Romesco is a great dip for green veggies and is traditionally served with asparagus. So yummy and healthy!

Ingredients:
- 2 tomatoes ripe, oven roast
- 1 whole head of garlic, oven roast
- 2 dried mild chili peppers, rehydrate in water (do it overnight)
- 12 almonds, blanch (or purchase raw almonds without skin)
- 15 hazelnuts blanch
- 1 cup olive oil (extra-virgin)
- 1/3 cup vinegar (red wine or sherry)
- 1 red pepper (roasted and either in a can or jar), drain
- A tiny bit of cayenne
- A pinch of Spanish paprika
- Salt to your liking

Instructions:
1. First the chilies must be rehydrated. Do this by covering them in water for as little as four hrs. or leave them all night. When they rehydrate, take out the seeds.
2. Roast your tomatoes. Peel them and set aside.
3. Roast your head of garlic, remove from the shell and set aside.
4. Peel your almonds/hazelnuts. (add nuts to boiling water for one minute, take out and rinse them under cold water right away to get skin off easily)
5. Put all ingredients into food processor or blender and blend well after they cool to room temperature.
6. Season with paprika, pepper and salt. Enjoy!

Tzaziki Spread/Dip

I love using this dip as a salad dressing (especially for salad with delicious olives and feta cheese!)

Ingredients:
- 3 garlic cloves
- 3 tbsp. fresh dill
- 1 cup cucumber
- 2 cups homemade/store bought Greek yogurt
- 1/2 tsp kosher salt
- 2 tbsp. fresh squeezed lemon juice
- 3 tbsp. olive oil

Instructions:
1. Throw everything into the blender or food processor and blend until creamy.
2. Put in the fridge for an hour or more.
3. Enjoy!

Use this versatile side as a sauce for baking, a dip for veggies and pita, or a spread! Both of these Greek sides would go well with a nice bottle of Athiri!

Delicious Greek Garlic Hummus

This super tasty and nutritious hummus can be used as a side dish, or a spread for your toasts. You can also enjoy it as a healthy snack, with some veggies!

Ingredients:
- 2 small garlic cloves
- 2.5 cup cooked chickpeas
- 1/2 cup tahini
- 1/2 tsp ground cumin
- 1/2 cup fresh lemon juice
- 3/4 tsp sea salt
- 3 tbsp. extra-virgin olive oil
- Dash of paprika
- A little extra olive oil to top

Instructions:
1. Allow chickpeas to soak overnight covered in water. They will double in size and loosen skins. Take off the skins, drain, add double the amount of water to more than cover and simmer for 1 ½ to two hours. Drain. Save the water.
2. Put the chickpeas into the food processor and pulse. Add tahini, lemon, and garlic, and pulse. Salt and cumin can be added now. Slowly add some of the cooked chickpea water and pulse until you reach desired consistency.
3. Put into a bowl, top with olive oil and paprika! So delicious!

Eat it on pita, whole grain crackers, fresh veggies, as a spread, or dilute 1:1 with water and stir with a fork to make a dressing! Other spices and roasted peppers can also be added. With hummus the options are pretty limitless.

Natural Banana Pudding

This recipe is naturally gluten and dairy free and it doesn't need sugar...It's naturally sweet!

Serves:4
Ingredients:
- 5 ripe bananas
- cup of rice milk (to be boiled) , half cup of rice milk (not to be boiled)
- tablespoons cornstarch (eco)
- tablespoon of agar-agar flakes
- a few drops of lemon essence (suitable for cooking)
- 1 tablespoon of apple juice concentrate
- 1 pinch of sea salt

Instructions:
1. Boil a cup of rice milk with agar-agar flakes until dissolved.
2. Peel and cut the bananas and put them in the bowl of the mixer. Add half cup of rice milk and the remaining ingredients. Whisk and when it is a creamy, add the rice milk with agar-agar (dissolved).
3. Finally, put the mix in molds. Garnish with strawberries, blueberries or kiwis and a little bit of cinnamon
4. Let it cool down a bit and put in the fridge.

This is one of my favorite snacks and desserts for the summer!

Part II

Recipes with Fish, Seafood and Meat

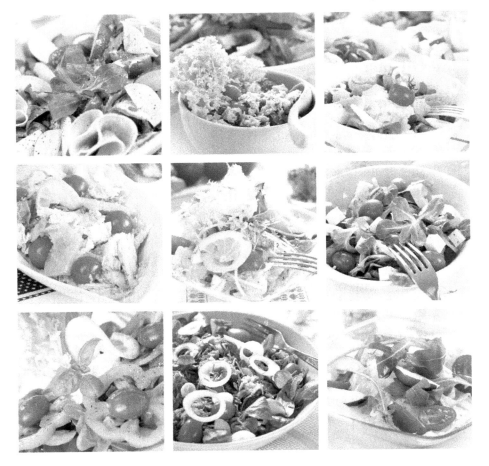

Simple Spanish Tuna Salad

This delicious recipe is low in carbs, abundant in clean protein, and high in nutrients. It's also very rich in good fats to help you stay full and energized for hours!

Serves: 3-4
Ingredients:
- 1 head of Romaine lettuce
- 2 rip roma tomatoes, cut into wedges (however big you like)
- 1 cucumber, peel and slice
- 1 can asparagus (white)
- 1 bell pepper, seed and slice into thin strips (lengthwise)
- 1 avocado, peeled, pit and slice
- ½ of a red onion, slice very thin
- 1 carrot, grate
- 2 hard-boiled eggs, peel and quarter (or trade for one can of albacore tuna in oil)
- red wine vinegar
- 2-4 tablespoons extra virgin Spanish olive oil
- salt (to your liking)
- 1 15 oz can artichoke hearts, drained

Instructions:
1. First, hard boil your two eggs. Then let them cool off in cold water and stick in freezer for a bit. When cool, peel and quarter.
2. Chop the whole romaine head in half and rinse and dry it.
3. Slice your tomatoes.
4. Slice cucumber after peeling.
5. Seed and the slice the peppers.
6. Grate carrot.
7. Open the cans of asparagus and artichokes and drain. Do the same if using tuna.
8. Tear up lettuce between two plates.
9. First lay on the tomato, then the cucumber, onion, pepper, and then carrots.
10. Break up the lettuce into small pieces for a salad. Make a bed of lettuce on a large platter. On top of the bed, place the tomatoes, cucumbers, onions, peppers and carrots. If using tuna spread it out around the lettuce.

11. Put the egg, asparagus, and artichoke on top.
12. Drizzle with oil and vinegar and salt to your liking.

Super Healthy Quinoa Pallea

This recipe is inspired by traditional Spanish paella, however, it uses quinoa instead of white rice, which makes this dish much more nutritious.

Serves: 2-4
Ingredients:
- 12-ounces of thawed shrimp (peel and devein)
- 2 carrots
- 2 turnips
- 12 asparagus, trimmed
- 2 young artichokes (make sure they are fresh)
- 1 lemon, cut in half
- 2 cup organic veggie broth
- ¼ cup extra virgin olive oil
- 2 cup scallions, slice very finely
- 2 garlic cloves, mince
- 1 ¼ cup quinoa
- 3 cup fresh peas
- 1 ¾ cup canned tomatoes (puree)
- ½ tsp of paprika (the sweet Spanish smoked variety is most authentic)
- Toast and pound ¼ tsp. saffron with a tad bit of salt.

Use a 13 ½ in. paella pan that you can put in the oven as well.

Instructions:

1. Rinse the carrots, turnips and asparagus and dry them.
2. Trim bottoms of the asparagus.
3. Trim artichoke as well.
4. Take the lemon halves and rub the artichokes with them. This will keep them from getting ugly. Put them aside in some lemon water.
5. Set your oven to 300.
6. Put the veggie broth in a separate pan and heat it up, but not to boiling.
7. Add evoo to the paella pan and turn the stove to medium. When hot, sauté turnips, asparagus spears, artichoke, carrot and onion for 2 min.
8. Put the garlic in the middle and cook for a few min. until all the veggies are soft and brown.
9. Now, put in the quinoa and continue sautéing until it turns clear. Do not let it get too brown.
10. Add your canned tomato puree and stir well. Add peas.
11. Let it thicken up and while scraping the pan at the bottom.
12. Next stir in the paprika and allow to cook for a couple more seconds.
13. Pour in the broth and add the shrimp. Mix it up very well. Allow it to boil. Now add the saffron and cook on high for about 15-17 min.
14. Put into the oven for 10-12 minutes.
15. Allow to set for 5 min and serve.
16. Enjoy! Goes great with a nice glass of Albariño.

Mediterranean Tuna Burger

This recipe is perfect for burger lovers! Why not enjoy a delicious burger in its healthier version? You can even serve it with one of the salads from this book! Total cooking and prep time for this recipe is about 1 hour (max), so be sure to try it when you have some more time to cook.

Serves: 4
Ingredients:
- 1 cup of fresh tuna
- 2 eggs
- clove garlic
- Some parsley
- Tomato
- Lettuce Hearts
- Turnips
- integral hamburger rolls
- Organic olive oil
- salt
- white pepper
- ketchup

Instructions:
1. Mash the tuna in a large bowl and add some minced garlic, chopped parsley, salt, pepper, and eggs. You can use a blender if you wish. Leave for about 30 minutes
2. In the meantime: peel, wash and cut the turnips into sticks.
3. Slice tomato and onion into rings.
4. Wash and slice the lettuce
5. Form the burgers from the tuna mixture. Fry.
6. Then, fry the turnip sticks in hot oil like potatoes.
7. Place the burgers on a hot plate with a drizzle of oil to make sure they remain juicy
8. Open the bread into two halves, add the burgers, sliced tomatoes and onions
9. Garnish with ketchup to taste.
10. Serve accompanied by fried turnips.

Mediterranean Chicken Flavored Veggie Soup

This soup is simple, tasty, nourish and fun. It uses organic chicken broth (you can also make your own) and combined it with vegetables to help you create optimal balance. This delicious soup is great to enjoy in winter or when you are looking for natural recipes to help you fight colds.

Serves: 4
Ingredients:
- 4 cups organic chicken broth
- 3 medium sweet potatoes
- 2 medium zucchinis
- 2 leeks
- piece of celery with leaves
- cloves of garlic
- Lemon juice (from 1 lemon)
- 1 tbsp. of fresh mint
- 1 tbsp. brown, cane sugar
- Ground white pepper
- Salt

OPTIONAL: I like adding carrots and broccoli to my soups to make them super detoxifying. If you have carrots and broccoli, add them to your soup with the zucchinis (the last step)

Instructions:
1. Peel the potatoes, rinse and cut.
2. Wash zucchini and cut into slices, without peeling.
3. Remove the green leaves of leeks, cut into slices, wash and drain.
4. Prepare celery. Peel and chop the garlic cloves.
5. Bring the broth to a boil in a saucepan and add the potatoes, leeks, celery, garlic, salt and a pinch of ground white pepper.
6. Add the lemon juice and sugar and simmer the broth for about 20 minutes.
7. Add the zucchini and mint and cook for 15 minutes.
8. Serve the soup hot.

Catalan "Pan Tomaquet"

Would you like to discover my traditional, juicy bread? This is actually a typical Catalan way of preparing "tomato bread".

It is great as a snack or aperitif. You can also serve it with salads and seafood.
Super quick prep time only 10 minutes

Serves: 4
Ingredients:
- loaf of gluten free, organic bread of your choice
- ripe tomatoes
- anchovies in brine
- Extra virgin olive oil
- Marine salt

Instructions:
1. Cut bread in small slices
2. Cut the tomatoes in halves; use them to run inside the bread so that it absorbs the juice and pulp of the tomato until completely red.
3. Smear the bread with a little bit of olive oil (not too much as the anchovies are already oily and salty)
4. Add the anchovies and enjoy!

OPTIONAL:
Apart from tomatoes, you can also use some garlic and rub it on your bread. It gives it a really nice taste! I also love adding some fresh rosemary! I love serving pan tomaquet with some tuna and sardines.

Traditional Salmorejo

This recipe is very similar to Spanish gazpacho but is a bit more complex. It is a really refreshing and energy providing dish, perfect for hot summers.

Serves:2
Ingredients:
- large ripe tomatoes
- 2 cloves of garlic
- 1 egg yolk (cooked)
- thick slice of organic bread
- Olive oil (about 2-3 tablespoons)
- tbsp. white wine vinegar
- Water
- Salt
- Half cup of organic ham (it can be also chicken or even seafood. I have also tried replacing meat with tofu, it's up to you which option you choose)
- boiled egg
- 1 small onion
- 1 green pepper

Instructions:
1. Peel the tomatoes and cut them.
2. Peel the garlic and cut into small pieces.
3. Moisten the bread with water.
4. Add: Garlic, egg yolk, tomatoes, olive oil and bread crumbs to a blender or a food processor.
5. Season with some salt and vinegar (about 2 tablespoons). Set aside to cool down in a fridge.
6. On a separate dish, prepare cut hum pieces, chopped hard-boiled eggs, and the rest of the ingredients you would like to see in your soup. Use your imagination.

<u>Rosemary Chicken</u>

This can be a nice family meal so make sure that everyone is involved in cooking! Rosemary chicken is just a classic in Spanish cuisine. Rosemary is actually the most popular herb used in Spanish cooking and was even dubbed "the queen of all herbs".

Serves:4
Ingredients:
- chicken 1.5 Kg (3.3 lb)
- lemon
- sprig of fresh rosemary
- half cup dry white wine
- 1 tbsp. olive oil
- pepper

Instructions:
1.Clean chicken. Wash and dry it.

2.Wash the lemon, dry it and insert it inside the chicken.

3.Arrange the chicken in a baking dish with 2 tablespoons of olive oil.

4.Sprinkle with chopped rosemary, put it in a preheated oven at 360 Fahrenheit (or 180 Celsius) and bake for 1 hour and 10 minutes. Turn over halfway through cooking.

5.Remove chicken from oven and retrieve the cooking juices (we will need it for the sauce).

6.Heat the wine in a saucepan and simmer for 2 minutes to reduce slightly. Then add the cooking juices and remove the sauce from heat. Serve chicken with this natural sauce.

Whole Wheat Pita Pockets

Whole wheat, home-made pita pockets can be a great addition to your vegetable soups and creams. Use them as a special treat!

Makes 8 servings
Ingredients:
- 3 ½ cup whole wheat flour
- 1 tbsp. active dry yeast
- ¼ cup water (warm)

Instructions:
1. Set oven to 500 degrees Fahrenheit (or 260 Celsius) and allow to preheat.

2. In a bowl, sift 2 cups of your flour with the yeast.

3. Once the dry ingredients are combined, mix in the water.

4. Add the other 1 ½ cups of flour slowly until the dough comes loose from the sides of the mixing bowl.

5. Now it is time to knead your dough. Knead well for four minutes.

6. Take out your dough and make it into eight evenly sized balls.

7. Flour a counter top or a large cutting board. Use a rolling pin and make each ball into a five or six in. circle. Do not roll them thinner than ¼ inch.

8. Spread some flour on each side of the pita.

9. Put each one on a non-stick cookie sheet and let them rise for a half hour.

10. Flip each one over carefully. Be sure not to pinch the edge or jostle them around too much.

11. Put them in the oven on the bottom rack and cook for five minutes, then remove.

12. After they are cool, place them in freezer zip-locks. Remove before using. They defrost very quickly!

13. When ready to use, slice them in half and fill! They can be re-warmed for a couple minutes in your oven at 350 degrees.

Delicious Greek Breakfast Pockets

This delicious recipe makes a perfect breakfast if you wake up hungry. It balances animal products with energy-boosting greens, like spinach.

Serves 2
Ingredients:
- 2 whole wheat pita pockets (home-made or bought)
- 6 egg whites
- 1/4 lb. turkey sausage (ground, 6 cut up links, or 3-4 patties)
- ½ tsp. chopped dill
- 1-2 cups spinach
- ½ tsp. each salt and pepper
- Greek yogurt (a dollop or two-recipe above) * optional

Instructions:
1. Cook the sausage in a frying pan according to directions.
2. Crack eggs, separate egg whites into a bowl, season, and whisk.
3. Add eggs to the cooked sausage in the same pan (draining grease first if you like) and cook over medium, stirring regularly for 3-5 min.
4. When eggs are almost done add spinach and dill. Allow it to slightly wilt and turn off the heat.
5. Add egg/sausage mixture to the pita pockets and throw in a dollop of Greek yogurt.
6. Serve with some fresh spinach!
7, Enjoy!

Greek Breakfast Shrimp on Toast

I am no a big meat person, but I love seafood! Also, usually, I just have a quick smoothie for breakfast. However, I love this recipe for special and family occasions.

Serves 4
Ingredients:
- 1/3 cup olive oil
- lb. shrimp (peel and de-vein)
- minced garlic cloves
- tomatoes (seed and chop)
- ½ bunch chopped green onion
- ½ c. feta (crumble)
- ½ of a lemon squeezed
- 1 tbsp. dry oregano
- 1 tsp dry thyme
- 1 tsp dry basil
- 1 tsp dry marjoram
- 1 tsp each dry onion and garlic (minced)
- Mix and store in airtight container.
- Greek loaf sliced (recipe above) into ½ in. slices

Instructions:
1. Place a large frying pan on the stove with 1 tablespoon oil and heat to medium high.
2. Add shrimp and garlic, sautéing for 4 min.
3. Remove from heat, place in a bowl, and chill.
4. Mix the tomatoes, 1 tablespoon olive oil, Greek seasoning, lemon juice, feta, and onion in another bowl and chill.
5. Take your bread slices and place them on a cookie sheet, brushing each one with olive oil. Place them in an oven set to 375 degrees Fahrenheit (or 190 Celsius) for 7-8 min.
6. When the bread is toasted, place some shrimp on each slice and top with tomato/cheese mixture.
7. Enjoy!

Delicious Balance Fish Frittata

This delicious recipe is also paleo and keto friendly. It fuses the revitalizing power of vegetables with quality animal products to help you create optimal balance.

Serves 4
Ingredients:
- free-range eggs
- 1 teaspoon pepper
- 1 teaspoon crushed red pepper
- Half teaspoon salt
- Any other seasonings of your choice
- 1 cup canned salmon
- ½ cup chopped bell pepper
- ½ cup chopped spinach
- ½ cup chopped kale

Instructions:
1. Set your oven to 350 degrees Fahrenheit (or 175 Celsius)
2. Grease a 9 in. pie or cake pan.
3. a bowl, whisk eggs, peppers, salt, and any other seasoning.
4. Place salmon and veggies in the bottom of your pan.
5. Now, carefully pour your eggs and seasonings over the fish and veggies.
6. Place the pan onto the middle rack in the oven for about 35 min. or until it is golden and firm.
7. Enjoy!

Halibut on Tomato Toast with Salad

This tasty recipe makes an excellent weekend dinner and goes really well with a big bowl of fresh salad.

Serves 6
Ingredients:
Toast
- 6 slices of thick crusty whole grain bread
- 4 cloves of garlic cut in half
- 3 ripe tomatoes cut in half
- Extra virgin olive oil
- Sea salt

Halibut
- ¼ c. fresh squeezed lemon juice
- ¼ cup extra virgin olive oil
- 4 cloves garlic (mince)
- 2 tablespoons paprika
- 2 tablespoons cumin
- 1 teaspoon salt
- ¼ tsp pepper
- 1 lbs. halibut filets (skinless)
- lemon (cut into 6 wedges)

Instructions:
1.In a mixing bowl, mix lemon, olive oil, minced garlic, paprika, half the salt and half the pepper.
2.Place fish in a baking dish. Marinate by rubbing marinade into both sides of the filets and allow to sit in fridge overnight.
3.Heat a grill or broiler. Season halibut with the rest of the salt and pepper. Cook for 3 minutes on each side.
4.Prepare toast.
5.Slice the bread and toast it.
6.Rub one side of toast with garlic.
7.Next, rub with tomato, while pushing down and squeezing in order to get pulp all over the toast.
8.Put one piece of toast on each place and top with halibut. Serve with lemon wedge. Serve sauce separately if desired.
9.Enjoy!

Egg-Lemon Tuna Soup

This recipe is original, tasty, nutritious and delicious. Tuna can make an amazing soup!

Serves 5-6
Ingredients:
- 3 carrots (chopped)
- 2 brown onions (chopped)
- 3-5 oz. cans tuna in oil (drained)
- 3 tablespoons fresh squeezed lemon juice
- ½ cup brown rice
- 5 cups vegetable broth (stock)
- 1 cup water
- 1 tbsp extra virgin olive oil
- Himalayan salt to taste
- 3 organic eggs

Instructions:
1. Cook brown rice according to the package.
2. While that is cooking, put a medium sized pot on the stove and heat oil to medium-high. Add onion and sauté for 5 minutes.
3. Add the veggie broth and the water to the cooked onions and simmer.
4. When the rice is finished, add the it to the onion broth, along with the drained tuna. Allow to simmer for 7 minutes.
5. In a separate bowl, whisk the eggs well. Add the lemon juice while continuing to whisk. Keep whisking until well blended.
6. Next, ladle in one full scoop of broth, still whisking constantly with the other hand. Repeat one more time.
7. Take the soup pot off of the heat and whisk as you add the egg/broth into the pot.
8. Enjoy!

Arugula Tuna with Lemon Parsley Dressing

This salad offers an incredible mix of clean protein, good fats, and superfood greens. The alkaline keto way!

Serves: 2
Ingredients
For the Salad:
- 1 whole scallion, finely chopped
- 2 cups of fresh arugula, chopped
- 1 avocado, peeled, pitted and sliced
- Fresh chopped parsley for topping
- 2 cans of organic tuna in olive oil

For the dressing:
- 4 tablespoons of thick coconut milk
- 4 tablespoons of parsley, chopped
- 2 tablespoons organic lemon juice
- 2 pinches of Himalayan salt (you can always add more if you need to)
- A pinch of black pepper and chili (optional)
- 1 big garlic clove, peeled

Instructions:
1. Combine all the salad ingredients in a big salad bowl and toss well.
2. Mix all the salad dressing ingredients using a small hand blender,
3. Pour the dressing over the salad and stir well.
5. Serve and enjoy!

Olive Green Veggie Salad

This salad is an excellent solution if you are looking for a meal replacing salad, something that will keep you full for many hours. It's a great mix of veggies, protein, and healthy, alkaline-keto fats!

Serves: 2
Ingredients
For the Salad:
- A few tablespoons of green olives
- 1 cucumber, peeled and finely chopped
- A few onion rings
- A handful of fresh baby spinach leaves
- 1 big garlic clove, peeled
- Half cup black olives pitted
- A few tomato slices
- A few almonds
- 2 cans of organic tuna

For dressing:
•2 tablespoons of organic Dijon mustard
•2 tablespoons of organic olive oil
•A few fresh basil and parsley leaves (optional)
•1 tablespoon of coconut vinegar
•Black pepper to taste

Instructions:
1. Combine all the salad ingredients in a big salad bowl and toss well.
2. Mix all the salad dressing ingredients. You can use a small hand blender, or quickly combine and stir all the ingredients in a small bowl.
3. Pour the dressing over the salad and toss well.
4. Sprinkle over a few mint, parsley, and cilantro leaves.
5. Serve and enjoy!

Grilled Chicken Salad with Grapefruit and Avocado

This keto-friendly dish is served with delicious alkaline fruits. It's perfect as a quick, comforting dinner recipe.

Serves:2-3
Ingredients
For the Salad:
- 4 skinless chicken breast halves (remove the bones)
- cups of mixed salad greens
- 1 cup of grapefruit chunks
- 3/4th cup of avocado, peeled and diced
- 3/4th teaspoon of grated fresh ginger

For the Dressing:
- 2 tablespoons of low carb mango chutney
- 2 tablespoons of olive oil
- 2 tablespoons of fresh lime juice
- 1 tablespoon of coconut aminos
- Cooking spray

Instructions:
1.Preheat a grill and grease it with some cooking spray.
2.Take a bowl and combine the coconut aminos, chutney, lime juice, olive oil, and ginger in it. Keep aside.
3.Lay the chicken breast halves on a flat surface and brush those with 2 tablespoons of the chutney mixture.
4.Grill the chicken for 4 minutes on each side while coating lightly with the chutney mixture again on flipping. Remove from grill once done.
5.Cut the chicken into diagonal pieces. Lay the avocado slices, grapefruit, and salad greens on the plate and place the chicken pieces on top to serve. Enjoy!

Simple Spicy Egg Scramble

This recipe is perfect as a tasty, energizing breakfast or a quick meal. Feel free to experiment with all kinds of spices for this one. Personally, I love chili powder!

Servings: 1-2
Ingredients:
- 2 tablespoons coconut oil
- Half cup shredded chicken
- 6 eggs
- 2 tablespoons coconut cream or thick coconut milk
- Pinch of chili powder
- Pinch of Pink Himalayan salt
- Pinch of freshly ground black pepper
- ½ cup shredded cheese
- Half cup green bell pepper, sliced
- A handful of chopped chive and dill

Instructions:
1. In a large skillet over medium-high heat, melt the coconut oil.
2. Add the chicken and sauté for 5 minutes until cooked.
3. In a separate bowl, whisk the eggs until frothy.
4. Now add the cream, salt, and spices.
5. Whisk to blend thoroughly.
6. Add the egg mixture to skillet with chicken and heat (on low heat) until almost cooked through, about 4 minutes.
7. When the eggs are almost done, add in shredded cheese and bell pepper.
8. Serve hot with some fresh chives and dill.

Turkey Broccoli Mix

This recipe proves how delicious and healing the alkaline keto mix can be.

Good fats, lean protein, and green veggies really help your body thrive and transform on a deeper level.

Servings: 2-3
* 6 turkey slices (thin)
* 1 small broccoli, cut into small florets, steamed or lightly cooked
* 4 garlic cloves, minced
* 1 small onion, diced
* 4 large eggs
* 2 tablespoon olive oil,
* Pink Himalayan salt
* Freshly ground black pepper

Instructions:
1. In a large skillet over medium-high heat, stir-fry the turkey slices in coconut oil (for about 2)
2. Turn the heat down to medium, and add the steamed broccoli florets, garlic, and onion.
3. Sautee for a few minutes.
4. When the veggies get tender, add the eggs by scrambling them all over the skillet. Keep stir frying until the eggs are set.
5. Sprinkle the olive oil on top, and serve hot.

Bonus – Alkaline Mediterranean Smoothie Recipes to Help You Look and Feel Amazing

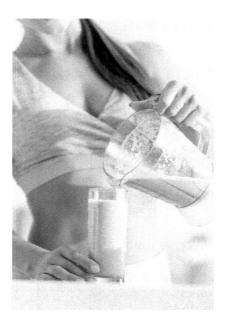

The following smoothie recipes are perfect if you are pressed for time. Some can be even served as a tasty and satisfying meal replacement!

Cucumber Dream Creamy Cheesy Smoothie

This is one of my favorite "on the go" smoothie recipes as it doesn't require that many ingredients.

It can also be transformed into a delicious raw soup.

I have created a fully plant-based version of this recipe which you can check out on the next page.

Servings: 2-3
Ingredients:
- 2 big cucumbers, peeled and roughly sliced
- 1 cup full-fat Greek Yoghurt
- 4 tablespoons grated goat cheese
- Pinch of Himalaya salt to taste
- Pinch of black pepper to taste
- 6 radishes, sliced
- 2 tablespoons chive, chopped

Instructions:
1.Place the cucumbers, and Greek Yoghurt in a blender.
2.Add the Himalaya salt and black pepper.
3.Blend well and pour into a smoothie glass or a small soup bowl.
4.Add in the radishes and chive.
5.Mix well and add more Himalaya salt and black pepper if needed. Sprinkle the cheese and enjoy!

Cucumber Dream Creamy Plant Based Alkaline Smoothie

This is a plant-based version of the previous recipe. It also tastes delicious, and I highly recommend it for days where your goal is detoxification to have more energy.

Servings: 2-3
Ingredients:
- 2 big cucumbers, peeled and roughly sliced
- 1 big avocado
- 1 cup of coconut milk
- 1 small lemon, peeled and sliced
- 4 tablespoons cashews, chopped or powdered
- Pinch of Himalaya salt to taste
- Pinch of black pepper to taste
- 6 radishes, sliced
- 2 tablespoons chive, chopped

Instructions:
1. Place the cucumbers, coconut milk, avocado and lemon in a blender.
2. Add the Himalaya salt and black pepper.
3. Blend well and pour into a smoothie glass or a small soup bowl.
4. Add in the radishes and chive.
5. Mix well and add more Himalaya salt and black pepper if needed. Sprinkle the cashews and enjoy!

Refreshing Radish Liver Lover Smoothie

Radish is a fantastic alkaline keto veggie that is very often overlooked. I always say there is no need to look for expensive and over-priced superfoods. Why not focus on what is already freely available? Radishes are very alkalizing and good for your liver and immune system. They are also very refreshing!

Servings: 1-2
Ingredients:
- Half cup radish, washed
- 1 small avocado, peeled and pitted
- A handful of fresh arugula leaves
- 1 cup full-fat coconut milk (no added sugar)
- Half cup of water
- Pinch of Himalaya salt to taste
- Pinch of black pepper to taste
- Optional: red chili pepper

Instructions:
1.Blend all the ingredients.
2.Serve in a smoothie glass or in a soup bowl- this smoothie can also be turned into a delicious soup.

If you serve this smoothie as a soup, feel free to add in some protein. It can be plant-based protein, for example, some nuts and seeds, or hard-boiled eggs. My husband loves to add in some smoked salmon or bacon.

Cilantro Oriental Alkaline Keto Smoothie

Cilantro is a miraculous alkaline herb with potent antioxidant properties. While making a curry can be very time-consuming, why not enjoy cilantro in a simple smoothie that you can make in less than 5 minutes).

Servings: 2-3
Ingredients:
- 2 cups coconut or almond milk
- 2 tablespoons coconut oil
- A handful of fresh cilantro leaves
- 1 small red bell pepper, sliced and seeded
- 1 teaspoon curry powder
- Pinch of Himalaya salt to taste
- Pinch of black pepper powder to taste

Instructions:
1. Combine all the ingredients in a blender.
2. Process until smooth.
3. Taste to check if you need to add more salt or spices.
Pour into a smoothie glass or a small soup bowl and enjoy!

Vitamin C Alkaline Keto Power

This delicious smoothie is jam-packed with vitamin C coming from alkaline and keto friendly fruits like limes and lemons. Now, I understand that looking at the ingredients of this recipe, you may be feeling a bit "turned off." Yes, alkaline keto smoothies are very different to usual "sweet fruity smoothies."

But, give it a try. It tastes great! Very similar to natural, Greek yogurt. You can also use this smoothie recipe to season your salads. Most salad seasonings are full of crappy carbs, sugars and a ton of chemicals, while this smoothie is 100% natural! Another suggestion is - you could use this smoothie recipe to make a smoothie bowl by adding in some nuts and seeds. Once you have tried this smoothie, you will get my point for sure!

Servings: 2
Ingredients:
- 1 big avocado, peeled, pitted and sliced
- Half lemon, peeled and sliced
- 1 cup of coconut milk
- 1 teaspoon coconut oil
- Pinch of Himalaya salt
- Pinch of black pepper
- A few slices of lime to garnish

Instructions:
1.Place all the ingredients in a blender.
2.Process until smooth.
3.Serve in a smoothie glass and garnish with a few lime slices.
4,Drink to your health and enjoy!

Hormone Rebalancer Natural Energy Smoothie

This smoothie recipe is a fantastic option if you don't like green smoothies, but you still want to experience all the health benefits of alkaline keto smoothies.

This recipe uses stevia which is a natural sweetener, very often used both on keto and alkaline diets.

Although, let me remind you that once your taste buds have adapted, you will be able to do without any sweeteners easily.
Still, if you need one- go for stevia.

Servings: 1-2
Ingredients:
- 1 big grapefruit, peeled and halved
- 1 cup water (filtered, preferably alkaline)
- 1 inch of ginger, peeled
- 1 tablespoon coconut oil
- Half teaspoon maca powder
- Stevia to sweeten, if desired

Instructions:
1.Blend all the ingredients in a blender.
2.Serve and enjoy!

Recommended Resources Mentioned in This Book

Alkaline Acid Charts available at:

www.YourWellnessBooks.com/charts

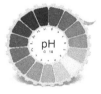

Alkaline Cleanse – discover how to lose weight and get rid of sugar cravings without feeling hungry or deprived:

www.YourWellnessBooks.com/cleanse

Sustainable weight loss after 40, 50, 60, and even 70…

www.YourWellnessBooks.com/weight-loss

Book 2 Paleo Salads

100+ Original Paleo Salad Recipes for Massive Weight Loss and a

Healthy Lifestyle

By Elena Garcia

INTRODUCTION

Dear Reader,

Thank you for taking interest in my book. I have written it to show you that eating a healthy Paleo-approved diet is not time-consuming at all. All you need to do is to get committed to it and decide to work on your creativity.

This recipe book is designed to help you become more creative and show you that Paleo salads are not only healthy and delicious but also exciting and fun to prepare.

This book is a great choice for everyone-yes everyone- no matter where you live, how old you are and what you do. Even if you are a vegan, you can benefit from this book, as I have also added a meat-free recipe section. The Paleo Diet is not only about consuming massive amounts of meat. I am not a scientist, but I believe that Paleo cavemen would eat whatever they could find. I am sure they would very often survive long periods of time just munching on fruit, nuts and veggies.

Here's my personal belief that you may agree or disagree with. Even though I am not a vegan or vegetarian, I really do try to eat less and less meat. I think it's healthier and better for the environment. Even if you are a Paleo fan, remember that there is much more to Paleo than just meat.

Of course, you can always change or customize my recipes. I include my e-mail in case you need me to lend you a hand or have problems finding ingredients or are allergic to any of them: elenajamesbooks@gmail.com

This book is especially recommended for:
-Paleo fans
-Alkaline Diet fans (everyone can benefit from adding more fresh fruit and veggies into their diets, right?)
-Health and wellness nuts
-Fitness enthusiasts
-People on weight loss regimes/programs
-Those who wish to detoxify and regain their wellness
-Those who are interested in low-carb diets

WHY I WROTE THIS BOOK

To be honest, I never thought I would write a Paleo recipe book. The reason is simple- I used to be really skeptical about Paleo. I am really passionate about healthy and balanced nutrition though and I love cooking. The diet that I really love (it helped me get healthy and lose weight) is the Alkaline Diet. I still maintain my healthy alkaline balance (70-80% alkaline foods) and I make sure everyone in my family gets used to greens and green smoothies.

However, I like variety as well. My number 1 rule is to go for organic, unprocessed foods and to listen to my body. I would also recommend getting fully committed to healthy cooking, it's not that difficult to learn, especially when it comes to salads.

Ok, so you must be thinking, why is this Alkaline green lady writing a Paleo book?

Well, I want Paleo people to discover more variety- fresh, nutritious, 100% Paleo friendly salad recipes. I also intend to get them hooked on fresh veggies and fruit!

The reason why I was skeptical about Paleo is that I imagined it was only about meat. Then, I began reading and researching and I realized that the true, healthy and balanced Paleo is very similar to the Alkaline Diet (not very strict one though). For example, you can reduce meat to 20% of your diet or even less and make the remaining 80% fresh, alkaline foods. That way you can be both Alkaline and Paleo. My husband and I wrote a bestselling book on how to do it (with practical steps and recipes) and if you are looking for more healthy and balanced nutritional ideas you will love the Alkaline-Paleo mix.

This book could be also approved by most Alkaline (non-vegetarian kind of alkalarians) people: the recipes are abundant in fresh fruit and veggies.

Both Alkaline Diet and Paleo Diet disapprove of bread (gluten products are not on the Alkaline Diet or Paleo Diet) and animal products like milk.

Here are the benefits of eating a Paleo Diet that is also abundant in alkalizing fruits and veggies:
You will detoxify your body and lose weight
You will improve your mental focus and concentrate better
You will restore your energy levels naturally, there will be no need to indulge in caffeine (topic for another book)
By eliminating gluten and processed foods as well as adding more fresh salads you will create a natural anti-inflammatory diet. As a result, your immune system will feel stronger doing a better job for you. Pain, inflammation, even headaches and PMS will be reduced.
Feeling skeptical?
I encourage you to do a little challenge- have at least 1 big bowl of salad a day. Salads are great for a quick-prep lunch. You can also make them to take to work. Fruit salads are a natural source of fiber and vitamins and a great way to reduce sugar cravings. Feeling like sugar? Go for a delicious, fruity, raw Paleo salad. This is going to be a much healthier treat! Plus your energy levels will skyrocket.

Ever since I switched to a natural, Paleo-Alkaline inspired approach and regained balance, I have been able to achieve my perfect weight without thinking too much about it. I don't know about you, but I found calorie counting pretty stressful.

There is also a bonus chapter where I show you how to make amazing, Paleo friendly salsas. Eliminating processed condiments is a must. I know many people who invest time and effort in buying organic greens, but they spoil all their work with artificial condiments.

Mini disclaimer:

Some ingredients suggested (like for example apple cider vinegar and other vinegars) are not Paleo, however many Paleo experts approve them in small amounts. It's up to you if you choose to do strick Paleo-Paleo, or modern Paleo (still healthy and natural).

By switching to natural, home-made salsas and other condiments, you will be able to save up money and make your salads more unique.

Happy salad-ing!

Enjoy!

Part 1 No Meat Paleo Salads

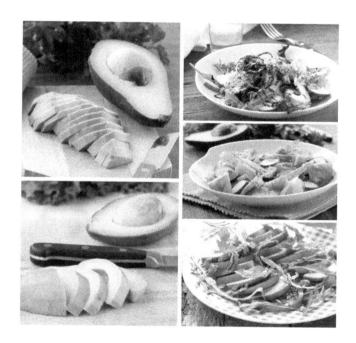

Thai Kale Salad

Servings: 6-7
Preparation time: 15-17 minutes
Cooking time: 2 minutes

Ingredients:

- 1½ lbs. (680 grams) of uncooked kale leaves, stemmed
- 1 large sized red onion, thinly sliced
- Coconut aminos (2 tablespoons)
- Juice of 2 limes
- ½ cup organic coconut milk
- 2 jalapeño peepers, diced
- Zest of 1 lime
- 2 orange sweet peppers, diced
- 3 cloves garlic, peeled, thinly sliced)
- Olive oil (about 2-3 tablespoons)

Method of preparation:

1.Sauté the red onion slices in some olive oil. Add the garlic clove, sweet peppers and jalapeño slices to the onions. Stir-fry until fragrant.

2.Blanch the kale leaves in a pot of boiling water for 2 minutes. Drain and set aside.

3.Mix the coconut aminos, lime zest and lime juice with the coconut milk. Set aside.

4.Toss the kale leaves with the sautéed vegetables and drizzle the coconut milk dressing on top to serve.

5.Enjoy!

Apple and Celery Root Salad

Servings: 2-3

Preparation time: 10-15 minutes

Cooking time: 2 hours

Ingredients:

- 1 medium red apple, (skin-on is optional), diced
- 2 tablespoons of Paleo mayonnaise*
- 1 medium sized celery root, peeled and grated
- 4 tablespoons of chopped walnuts
- Paleo Gremolade (2 teaspoons)
- Juice of 1 lemon
- 2 fresh scallions, sliced
- 2 tablespoons of coconut cream
- 1/4th cup of minced fresh parsley leaves

Method of preparation:

1.Toss celery root with diced apples and lemon juice. Then add-in the scallions, walnuts and parsley. Toss again to combine.

2.Mix the gremolade and mayonnaise with coconut yoghurt in another bowl.

3.Add the mayonnaise salad dressing to the apples mixture and then toss to combine.

4.Cover the salad bowl with saran wrap. Store in a fridge for a couple of hours. Serve chilled.

*How to make Paleo Mayo (non-vegan option)

Mix: 1 egg yolk with a pinch of Himalaya salt, half teaspoon of Dijon mustard, 1 tablespoon of lemon juice and a few drops of white vinegar and half cup of avocado oil or coconut oil. Enjoy!

*How to make Paleo Mayo (vegan option)

Mix: half cup almond or coconut milk, 2 tablespoons fresh lemon juice, 1 tablespoon Dijon mustard, half cup of olive oil, pinch of salt and pepper. You can experiment with the consistency by adding some almond powder and coconut oil. Enjoy!

Really Simply Kale Caesar Salad with Artichoke Hearts and Pickled Red Onions

Servings: 4-5

Preparation time: 10 minutes

Ingredients:

- 2-3 brine dipped artichoke hearts, halved
- 2 cups of fresh kale leaves, stemmed and coarsely chopped
- Half cup of almond powder mixed with cashew powder (our vegan "parmesan cheese")
- 1 pickled red onion, sliced

Ingredients for the Caesar Dressing:

- 2/3rd cup of homemade mayonnaise (paleo) (check the recipe from the previous recipes)
- 1 garlic clove, peeled and minced
- 6 whole anchovy filets
- Olive oil (3 tablespoons)
- Juice of 1 big lemon

Method of preparation:

1.Mix all the salad ingredients in a big bowl. Set aside.

2.Blend all the ingredients for the salsa.

3.Mix with the salad, stir well and enjoy!

Samphire Roast Lemon and Hazelnut Salad

Servings: 2-3
Preparation time: 10-15 minutes
Cooking time: 20 minutes

Ingredients:
- 1 oz. (180 grams) of Samphire
- Organic maple syrup, (2 teaspoons)
- 0.881 oz. (25 grams) of hazelnuts
- 1 whole lemon, sliced
- 3 whole radishes
- Olive oil (about 2 tablespoons)

SALAD SALSA
- 1 tablespoon of maple syrup
- 2 tablespoons olive oil,
- Fresh juice of half a lemon
- 2 tablespoons of finely chopped fresh mint leaves

Method of preparation:
1.Preheat an oven to 446 degrees Fahrenheit. Slice lemon into thin slices.
2.Mix the olive oil with the maple syrup (use a bowl). Dip the lemon slices in the maple syrup mixture. Then put on a parchment paper lined baking tray.
3.Insert the tray in the oven and roast for 20 minutes or until the lemon slices start to brown.
4.Mix olive oil, maple syrup and lemon juice. Whisk well to combine and then add-in the mint leaves to prepare the dressing.
5.Lay the hazelnuts in a baking tray and roast for 5 minutes. Steam the samphire for 1 minute over a steamer in the meantime and then rinse the leaves under cold water. Drain properly and set aside. Finally, toss the steamed samphire leaves with the roasted lemon slices and hazelnuts. Drizzle the seasoning on top and to serve. Enjoy!

Carpaccio of Summer Veggies

Servings: 4
Preparation time: 20-30 minutes

Ingredients:
- 1 red organic beetroot, peeled and sliced
- 6 whole radishes, sliced
- 1 orange beetroot, peeled and sliced
- 1/2 of a red onion, peeled and sliced
- 2 small courgettes, (zucchini) sliced
- 1 small sized kohlrabi, sliced
- 1 red pepper, deseeded and sliced
- ¼ cup of almonds

Dressing:
- 3 fl. oz. (90 ml) of olive oil (extra virgin)
- 2 teaspoons of fresh oregano, chopped
- 1 clove of garlic, peeled and finely chopped
- 1 teaspoon of organic maple syrup
- 1 tablespoon of fresh parsley leaves, chopped
- 1 tablespoon of water
- Fresh juice of 1 lemon
- Sea salt (a pinch)

Method of preparation:
1.To make the dressing, whisk 3 fl.oz. of olive oil with water, 1 clove of chopped garlic and maple syrup. Then add lemon juice, sea salt, parsley and oregano. Whisk again to combine. Set aside in a fridge while you are preparing the salad.
2.Mix the sliced veggies in a big bowl. Add some almonds and drizzle the salad dressing on top to serve the salad.

Green Papaya Salad

Servings: 2
Preparation time: 15 minutes

Ingredients:
- 1.763 oz. (50g) of mixed fresh lettuce leaves
- ½ of a green papaya, julienned
- 1 whole radish, sliced
- ½ of a small carrot, julienned
- 2 tablespoons of raw cashew nuts
- A few whole cherry tomatoes, quartered

For the Chilli Spicy Dressing:
- 1 tablespoon of raw coconut vinegar
- 1 tablespoon of raw organic honey
- 2 tablespoons of water
- 1 red long chili, seeded and finely chopped
- Juice of 2 limes
- ½ tablespoon of paleo fish sauce (optional but I suggest you give it a try)
- 1 small clove of garlic, peeled and minced

Method of preparation:
1.Toss the julienned carrots and papaya with radish and lettuce leaves. Transfer the carrots to a salad bowl.

2.Top with the quartered cherry tomatoes and cashews. Set aside.

3.In a separate bowl take the chili slices and other dressing ingredients listed above. Whisk to combine. Set aside in a fridge (optional- depends on your time really)

4.Now mix the salad with the dressing so that all ingredients are equally covered. Serve with some lemon wedges. Enjoy!

Grilled Zucchini Salad

Servings: 4
Preparation time: 15-20 minutes
Cooking time: 10-12 minutes

Ingredients:
- 4 whole fresh zucchini, quartered lengthwise
- 1.5 cup of cherry tomatoes, quartered or halved
- 2 tablespoons of sweet onion, minced
- 2 teaspoons of olive oil (extra virgin)
- kalamata olives, pitted and roughly chopped
- A pinch of crashed garlic
- 1 tablespoon of fresh lemon thyme
- 1 tablespoon of fresh dill, chopped
- 1 teaspoon of Dijon mustard (optional)
- Pinch of Himalaya salt
- 1/4th teaspoon black pepper
- Juice from 1/2 a lemon
- 1-2 tablespoons of avocado oil
- Sea salt, according to taste
- Black pepper, to taste

Method of preparation:
1.Toss the zucchini quartered slices in 2 teaspoons of olive oil, salt, garlic, and a bit of black pepper.
Set aside and allow the zucchini slices to marinade for 10 minutes.
2.Grill over medium heat once marinating is done until the zucchini slices are charred a bit.
3.Remove from grill once done and let it cool down.
4.Slice the zucchini and set aside.
5.In the meantime, mix some olive oil with mustard and lemon juice.
6.You can mix them directly in a big bowl.
7.Add the cherry tomatoes, olives and sweet onion slices to the zucchini and then toss the vegetables with the olive oil mustard mixture you have just prepared. I sometimes throw in a few raisins, but this is optional.
8.Finally add the chopped herbs and toss again. Serve and enjoy!

Summer Slaw with Tahini Coconut Dressing

Servings: 4
Preparation time: 30 minutes
Cooking time: 10-15 minutes

Ingredients for slaw:
- 1 head of fennel, cored and sliced
- 1/4th cup of raisins
- 1/4th of a head of purple cabbage, cored and sliced
- 1/4 cup of Thai basil
- 1 whole bell pepper (yellow colored), seeded and sliced

Ingredients for the dressing:
- 2 tablespoons of fresh coconut milk
- 2 tablespoons of paleo tahini
- 1 inch of fresh ginger, grated (you can also use 1-2 teaspoons of ginger powder)
- 1 teaspoon of paleo raw honey
- Juice of 1 lime
- Pinch of Himalaya Salt
- Pinch of Black pepper

Ingredients for curried cashews:
- 1 cup of raw cashew nuts
- 1/4th teaspoon of paprika
- 1 tablespoon of raw coconut oil
- 1 tablespoon of lime juice
- 1 ½ teaspoons of paleo curry powder
- 1/4th teaspoon of chili powder
- 1/4th teaspoon of turmeric powder

Method of preparation:
1. To prepare the cashews, heat up 1 tablespoon coconut oil in a pan and add the lemon juice and herbs to the oil. Stir fry for a minute and then drop the cashews in the oil.

2. Stir the nuts in the oil for a minute and transfer to a parchment paper lined cookie sheet.

3.Bake the nuts in a 350 degrees preheated oven for 10-15 minutes or unless the nuts turn golden brown in color and crispy. Remove once done and let cool. To prepare the slaw, toss the chopped fennel with cabbage, basil leaves and yellow pepper slices. Whisk all the added ingredients needed to prepare the dressing until a smooth dressing is formed. Drizzle the dressing over the salad and drop the raisins and cashew nuts on top to serve.

Beet Salad with Toasted Almonds

Servings: 4

Preparation time: 5-10 minutes

Cooking time: 1 hour

Ingredients:

- 4 whole cooked beets, peeled and sliced
- 1/2 cup of cashew powder
- 2 cups of frisee
- 1 tablespoon of coconut oil
- 1 large apple, cored and sliced thinly
- 1/4th cup olive oil
- tablespoons of almonds
- Sea salt or Himalaya salt to taste

Method of preparation:

1.Boil the beets after trimming their heads. Once boiling, reduce the heat and simmer for about half an hour. Once done, drain and transfer the beets to sink and let sit under cold running water.

2.Once cold, peel off skins of beets and chop into bite sized pieces.

3.Toast the almonds over medium heat for 5 minutes in coconut oil; set aside.

4.Take the beets in a salad bowl and add the frisee, toasted almonds and apple slices. Toss well.

5.Finally toss with sea salt and olive oil. Serve with powdered cashews.

Raw Broccoli Slaw

Servings: 4
Preparation time: 10-15 minutes
Cooking time: 10-15 minutes

Ingredients:

- Shredded carrots (1 cup)
- ½ cup of fresh red cherries
- 1½ cups of broccoli florets, shredded
- 3/4th cup of red cabbage, shredded
- ½ cup of thinly sliced red onion
- 1 cup of baby kale leaves

Dressing:

- 3 teaspoons of chia seeds
- 3 teaspoons of Dijon mustard
- 6 tablespoons of coconut vinegar
- 6 tablespoons of extra virgin olive oil
- 1/4th cup of raw honey
- 1/4th teaspoon of freshly crackled black pepper
- ½ teaspoon of koshersalt

Method of preparation:

1.Process the carrots and broccoli florets in a food processor to shred those. Transfer to a large sized salad bowl.

2.Add the onion slices, cherries, kale leaves and shredded red cabbage.

3.Prepare the dressing by mixing everything in a separate bowl.

4.Drizzle the dressing over the slaw and toss before serving.

Rainbow Salad

Servings: 4-5

Preparation time: 10-15 minutes

Ingredients:

- 1 whole cucumber, diced without peeling
- 1 teaspoon of Dijon mustard (optional)
- 3/4 cup of purple cabbage, chopped
- ½ teaspoon of onion powder
- 1 tablespoon of coconut vinegar
- 2 teaspoons of raw organic honey
- 1 medium sized ripe tomato, diced
- 1 teaspoon of dill
- A pinch of garlic sea salt
- A pinch of ground black pepper

Method of preparation:

1.Chop the vegetables (cabbage, tomato and cucumber) and mix in a bowl.

2. the dressing and mix well.

3.Serve the salad right away.

<u>Creamy Yummy Broccoli Salad</u>

Servings: 4-6
Preparation time: 20-25 minutes

Ingredients:

- 4 cups of broccoli florets, chopped and steamed
- 1/2 cup of green olives, sliced
- 1/4 cup of pecans, chopped
- 2 mini seedless cucumbers, peeled and diced
- Half cup of raisins
- 4 tablespoons raw coconut vinegar
- 4 cups chopped baby spinach leaves
- 1/2 cup of paleo homemade mayonnaise of your choice (check the previous recipes)
- Juice of 1/2 a lemon
- 1 yellow bell pepper, finely chopped
- 1 orange bell pepper, finely chopped
- 1/2 of a red apple, julienned
- 1 whole red bell pepper, finely chopped
- 1/4 teaspoon of Himalayan salt
- 1/2 teaspoon of black pepper
- 2 slices of lemon or lime to garnish

Method of preparation:

1.Chop the broccoli florets, bell peppers, baby spinach leaves, green olives and cucumbers and set aside in a bowl. Add the rest of the ingredients.

2.Finally sprinkle over the dressing and stir well. Season with salt and pepper to taste.

3.Garnish with a slice of lime or lemon.

4.Enjoy!

Spaghetti Squash Yoga Bowl

Servings: 4
Preparation time: 20 minutes
Cooking time: 10 minutes

Ingredients:
- 2 bunches of small broccoli
- 2 lbs. (907 grams) of spaghetti squash
- 1 tablespoon of coconut oil
- 4 kale stalks
- Cashew nuts
- Sesame seeds
- Red pepper flakes

Sauce:
- Coconut aminos (2 tablespoons)
- 2-3 medium garlic cloves
- 1 tablespoon of coconut sugar
- 1 tablespoon of coconut vinegar
- 2 tablespoons raw cashew butter
- 1 1-inch piece of fresh ginger, peeled and grated
- 1/3 cup coconut oil
- 1 whole lime
- 1/2 tablespoon of Himalaya salt
- 1 tablespoon of sesame oil

Method of preparation:

1.Cook the spaghetti squash until thoroughly cooked. Remove the spaghetti squash from the heat and let it cool down.

2.Scrape and extract the flesh of the squash.

3.To prepare the sauce for the salad, process all the sauce ingredients in a food processor.

4.Process to get a smooth salad sauce. Set the sauce aside in a bowl once done.

5.Toss the spaghetti squash with the salad sauce and set aside.

6.Chop the broccoli florets and set those aside in a bowl.

7.Heat up 1 tablespoon of coconut oil in a skillet and stir-fry the broccoli florets. Keep stir-frying until slightly brownish.

8.Then add the kale leaves and cook those for a few more minutes. Make sure the kale leaves start to wilt. Finally add-in the spaghetti squash and cook for a few more seconds until cooked through.

9.Serve the salad with cashew nuts, red pepper flakes or sesame seeds. Enjoy!

Spinach Almonds and Tomatoes Salad

Servings: 4

Preparation time: 10-15 minutes

Cooking time: 15-20 minutes

Ingredients:

- 1/2 cup of almonds
- 2 cups of baby spinach
- 2 big carrots, peeled and sliced
- 15 cherry tomatoes
- 1 teaspoon of red chili flakes
- 2 teaspoons of sumac
- 2 medium garlic cloves (peeled and chopped)
- 1 tablespoon of olive oil
- A pinch of Himalaya sea salt

Method of preparation:

1.Toast the almonds in some olive oil. Stir to mix and set aside to allow it to cool down the almonds.

2.Then, stir-fry the garlic and red pepper. Add the tomatoes once the garlic is slightly browned. Cook until the tomatoes start releasing their juices.

3.Finally add the sumac and the toasted almonds to the tomato mixture. Stir the mixture to combine well. Cool it down and mix with spinach and carrots. Store in a fridge for about 15 minutes. Add a bit of Himalaya salt and olive oil to taste. Serve and enjoy!

Salad Savoy

Servings: 4-5
Preparation time: 15-20 minutes
Cooking time: 15-17 minutes

Ingredients:
- ½ cup of shiitake mushrooms
- 1 bunch of salad savoy cabbage
- 2 tablespoons of vegan cheese (powdered almonds and cashews)
- 1 medium sized red onion, peeled and sliced
- 1 medium sized clementine, peeled and segmented
- 2 cloves garlic (peeled, minced)
- 4 stalks of asparagus, cut into ribbons
- 1 tablespoon of coconut butter

Ingredients for dressing:
- 1 lemon, juiced
- Sea salt, to taste
- 2 tablespoons of olive oil
- A dash of grated ginger

Method of preparation:
1.Melt the coconut butter in a skillet and dump the onion and garlic slices to the oil.
2.Sauté the onions and garlic until softened and translucent in color. Once that happens, add the asparagus ribbons and shiitake mushrooms to the onion mixture in the skillet.
3.Then add the salad savoy to the mixture and cook the mushrooms mixture lid-on on low heat for 5 minutes.
4.Remove the lid from the skillet, give stir the mixture lightly and cook the mixture again without lid for 10 minutes on low heat.
5.Finally add the vegan Paleo cheese and the clementine segments to the salad. Give a nice stir to combine, turn down the heat and let it cool down a bit.
6.In the meantime, blend all the salad ingredients.
7.Toss the salad with the dressing and serve right away. Enjoy!

Simple Celery Salad

Servings: 2-3

Preparation time: 10 minutes

Ingredients:

- 1 ½ cups of celery, sliced

- 1 ½ tablespoons of Paleo mayonnaise

- 1 tablespoon of chives (minced)

- 1/2 teaspoon of fresh, organic lemon juice

- Sea salt, to taste

- 3 tablespoons raw raisins

- A pinch of black pepper

Method of preparation:

1.Stir and mix the paleo mayonnaise with lemon juice, sea salt and black pepper using in a salad bowl.

2.Slice the celery and chives. Dump the sliced vegetables and the raisins in the mayonnaise mixture.

3.Stir and toss the salad to coat the vegetables with the mayonnaise dressing and then serve to enjoy.

Pistachio Kale Salad

Servings: 4
Preparation time: 20-30 minutes

Ingredients:
- ½ cup of shelled pistachios, roughly chopped
- 2 bunches of dinosaur kale, very thinly sliced
- 4 scallions, very thinly sliced
- ¼ cup of raw sesame seeds

For the salad:

- 1/3 cup of paleo tahini paste
- 1/3 cup of plain water
- 1 garlic clove, peeled
- Sea salt, to taste
- 2 tablespoons of juice of lemon
- 1 tablespoon miso paste

Method of preparation:

1.To prepare the salad dressing, blend all the ingredients until smooth and lightly thick. Add more water or coconut milk to the salad dressing to achieve the right consistency.

2.Cut and chop the vegetables and combine the kale with scallions in a bowl. Pour the salad dressing over the scallion mixture and toss to combine.

3.Finally, sprinkle the sesame seeds and the chopped pistachios on top of the salad to garnish and serve the salad

Greek Style Bell Pepper Salad

Servings: 4
Preparation time: 20-25 minutes

Ingredients:

- 1 large orange bell pepper (cut into chunks)
- 1 cup of jumbo Kalamata olives, pitted
- 1 large yellow bell pepper (cut into chunks)
- 2 green onions, chopped
- 1 green bell pepper, cubed
- 1/2 cup of organic walnuts, chopped
- 1 red bell pepper, cut into chunks
- 4 medium Lebanese cucumbers, halved lengthwise, seeded and sliced
- 1/4 cup parsley
- 1/2 lb. (225 grams) of paleo cashew feta cheese, diced

***To make Paleo Cashew Feta Style Cheese, simply blend the following ingredients: 1 cup of raw cashews previously soaked in water for at least a few hours (I leave it to soak overnight and I use alkaline water), about ¼ cup of almond milk or coconut milk, 1 tablespoon of lime juice, ¼ cup of nutritional yeast, 1 clove of garlic and a bit of Himalaya salt to taste. Transfer into little cubes (like for ice making) and store in a fridge for a few hours.

Ingredients for the vinaigrette:

- 1 tablespoon of za'atar
- 1/4th cup of olive oil (extra-virgin)
- 1 tablespoon of dried oregano, organic
- 2 tablespoons of paleo vinegar (white wine)
- 2 large garlic cloves, peeled and minced
- 1/2 teaspoon of Himalayan salt
- 1 tablespoon of sumac
- 1/2 teaspoon fresh black pepper

Method of preparation: Prepare the salad dressing by taking all the ingredients required for the vinaigrette in medium sized bowl. Whisk with a fork or a blender to prepare the dressing. Now peel and chop all the vegetables and transfer to a salad bowl. Drizzle the homemade vinaigrette over the salad. Toss lightly to coat the vegetables with the vinaigrette. Serve the salad as it is or chill for a few hours before serving.

<u>Gingered Peas and Cucumber Salad</u>

Servings: 5

Preparation time: 10 minutes

Ingredients:

- 3 Persian cucumbers, peeled and thinly sliced

- 1 tablespoons of grated ginger

- 2 tablespoons of olive oil

- 1 teaspoon of raw honey

- 2 tablespoons of pure organic lemon juice

- 1 shallot, thinly sliced

- Zest of 1 lemon

- Black pepper, to taste

- Sea salt, to taste

Method of preparation:

1.Slice the shallots and cucumbers. Set aside the chopped vegetables in a salad bowl.

2.Now combine the lemon zest, grated ginger, lemon juice, black pepper, olive oil and sea salt. Mix well and add to the salad. Serve right away. Enjoy!

Cucumber and Radish Salad

Servings: 5-6

Preparation time: 20-25 minutes

Ingredients:

- 1 whole cucumber, thinly sliced

- 3 stems of parsley leaves, stemmed and chopped

- whole radishes, sliced thinly

- Sea salt, to taste

- 2 tablespoons raw coconut vinegar

- ½ of a red onion, peeled and sliced thinly

- 2 tablespoons of olive oil

- Black pepper, to taste

Method of preparation:

1.Slice the radishes, cucumber and onion. Set aside the sliced vegetables in a bowl.

2.Remove the leaves from the parsley stems and add those to the sliced vegetables in the bowl.

3.Now add the coconut vinegar, sea salt, olive oil and ground black pepper to salad. Mix well. Enjoy!

SECTION 2 FISH-Y PALEO SALADS

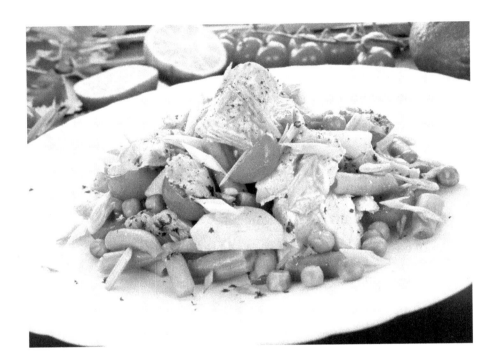

__Two Minutes Tuna Salad__

It takes only a couple of minutes to prepare, but you need much more time to drool over it!

Servings: 2-3

Preparation time: 2-3 minutes

Ingredients:

- 1 can of paleo albacore tuna, drained

- 2 tablespoons of cashew nuts

- 1/4 cup of chopped tomatoes

- 2 cups of baby spinach

- 2-3 tablespoons of homemade paleo pesto (simply blend some olive oil with Himalaya salt and fresh basil leaves and tomato juice)

- 1/4 cup of chopped bell peppers

Method of preparation:

1.Take drained tuna in a bowl. Add the bell peppers, spinach, cashew nuts and tomatoes to the tuna.

2.Toss the drained tuna mixture with pesto. Serve.

3.Enjoy!

Confetti Rice Salad with Salmon

Servings: 2

Preparation time: 5-10 minutes

Ingredients:

- 1 cup of steamed cauliflower rice
- 3-4 oz. (113.4 grams) of cooked salmon
- 1/3rd cup of artichoke hearts
- 4 teaspoons of paleo mayonnaise
- 2 teaspoons of toasted cashew nuts
- 4 teaspoons of paleo white balsamic vinegar
- 1 cup celery, finely sliced
- 1 teaspoon of extra virgin olive oil
- 1/3rd cup of thinly sliced red or orange bell peppers
- 1/4th teaspoon of dry thyme
- 1.5 teaspoons of curry powder
- 11 whole scallion, sliced
- A pinch of Himalaya salt
- Fresh ground black pepper, according to taste

Method of preparation:

1.Whisk together thyme, paleo mayonnaise, balsamic vinegar, curry powder, olive oil and a pinch of salt. Set aside.

2.Add the scallions, artichoke hearts, bell pepper slices, celery slices, salmon and cashews with the cauliflower rice.

3.Add the mayonnaise dressing and toss again before serving to make sure it's equally spread on all the ingredients. Enjoy!

<u>Apple Pecan Tuna Salad</u>

Servings: 2-3

Preparation time: 10 minutes

Ingredients:

- 1 can of drained tuna
- 3 tablespoons of pecans
- 1/2 an apple, diced
- 1-2 tablespoons coconut yogurt
- 1/2 a stalk of celery, diced
- Ground black pepper, as required
- 1/2 lemon, juiced
- Sea salt, to taste

Method of preparation:

1.Chop the fruits and vegetables as is instructed and put in a bowl.

2.Add the remaining ingredients and stir well to combine. Serve and enjoy! I love coconut yoghurt or coconut milk (a nice alternative if you can't find coconut yoghurt) in my salads!

Quick Salmon Salad

Servings: 2-3
Preparation time: 10-15 minutes

Ingredients:

- 1 can of wild caught salmon, drained
- 1/4 cup of radicchio, shredded
- 1/4 cup of raw walnuts, chopped
- 1/2 ripe avocado (peeled and diced)
- 3.5oz. (100g) mixed leafy greens
- 4 tablespoons of paleo mayo
- 1 medium sized endive, sliced
- 3 oz. (85g) of baby spinach leaves, roughly chopped
- 2 tablespoons of lemon juice
- 3 large sized mushrooms, stemmed and sliced
- 1 small seedless cucumber, diced
- 1/2 teaspoon of freshly cracked black pepper
- 1 teaspoon of herbes de Provence
- 1/4 teaspoon of Himalayan or sea salt
- 2 tablespoons of olive oil

Method of preparation:

1.Dump everything into a salad bowl after chopping and slicing as necessary. Mix well.

2.Season the salad with Himalayan salt, pepper, olive oil, lemon juice and toss well to combine.

3.Sprinkle the remaining salmon on top to serve.

Creamy Tarragon Tuna Apple Salad

Servings: 2
Preparation time: 10 minutes

Ingredients:

- 2 small sized cans of wild tuna
- 1/2 of an English cucumber, peeled and finely chopped
- 1 whole apple, cored and chopped
- Honeyed Walnuts (optional)
- 2 whole scallions, minced

Ingredients for dressing:

- 4 tablespoons of paleo mayo
- 3 tablespoons of tarragon, minced
- 1 small clove of garlic
- Sea salt, to taste
- 1 tablespoons of fresh lemon juice
- Pinch of black pepper

Method of preparation:

1.To prepare the salad, empty the tuna can into a large salad bowl. Add the remaining ingredients and stir well to combine.

2.Prepare the dressing by mixing the ingredients for the dressing in a separate bowl.

3.Pour the salad dressing over the salad, toss lightly and serve. Enjoy!

Salmon Arugula Salad with Lemon Parsley Dressing

Servings: 4
Preparation time: 40 minutes

Ingredients:

- 1 lb. (453 g) of grilled salmon fillets
- 1 whole scallion, finely chopped
- 4 cups of fresh arugula, chopped
- Fresh chopped parsley for topping
- 1 whole ripe avocado, peeled, pitted and cubed
- 2 tablespoons of capers (optional)

For the dressing:

- 2 tablespoons of extra virgin olive oil
- 4 tablespoons of parsley, chopped
- 2 tablespoons organic lemon juice
- Sea salt
- A pinch of pepper
- Lemon wedges, for garnishing

Method of preparation:

1.Cut the cooked or grilled salmon filets into bite sized pieces and place in a bowl.
2.Chop the vegetables as mentioned.
3.Combine everything with the salmon pieces except for the fresh parsley. Toss to mix and transfer the bowl to a refrigerator to let the salad sit there for 30 minutes.
4.In the meantime, prepare the salad dressing by mixing all the salad dressing ingredients (use a small bowl). Set aside.
5.Once the salad is cooled down, drizzle the dressing on top.
6.Toss the salad to mix the dressing and then finally sprinkle fresh parsley on top to serve. Enjoy!

Poached Cod and Citrus Salad

Servings: 2

Preparation time: 8-10 minutes

Cooking time: 4-5 minutes

Ingredients:

- 2 fresh filets of cod
- Juice of 1 lemon
- 1 whole fennel bulb with the stalks
- 1/2 tablespoons of olive oil
- 1/2 teaspoon of fennel leaves
- 1 medium-sized sweet tangelo or orange or blood orange, peeled and sliced
- A pinch of sea salt

Method of preparation:

1.Bring a pot of water to boil. In the meantime, cut the fennel bulb into thin slices. Set aside.

2.Mix the olive oil with fennel leaves, sea salt and lemon juice. Set aside.

3.Once water starts boiling, drop the cod filets in the water and poach for 4-5 minutes until the filets turn opaque and flaky in nature. Cool to cut into bite sized pieces.

4.Slice the citrus fruit after peeling it. Slice the fruit horizontally to get wheel-like slices.

5.Toss the fennel bulb slices with citrus slices and cod pieces. Drizzle lemon juice dressing on top and toss again to serve. Enjoy!

Keto Tuna Salad

Servings: 2-3

Preparation time: 5 times

Cooking time: 8-10 minutes

Ingredients:

- 1 3.5-oz. (100g) head of lettuce, (Little Gem or Romaine)
- 2 tablespoons of paleo mayonnaise (preferably homemade)
- 6oz. (180g) of organic tuna, drained
- Juice from 1/4th of a lemon
- 2 hard-boiled eggs, free-range
- A bit of olive oil
- 1 0.5-oz. (15g) medium sized spring onion
- Himalayan salt, to taste

Method of preparation:

1.Hard boil the eggs and then cut those in halves. Line salad bowl with the lettuce leaves.

2.Place the egg halves all over the lettuce leaves, so as to place an egg half over one lettuce leaf. Toss the tuna pieces in the lemon juice before placing over the lettuce leaves.

3.Drizzle the mayonnaise and extra virgin olive oil over the salad and serve.

Nicoise Salad

Servings: 2-3
Preparation time: 20 minutes
Cooking time: 15-20 minutes

Ingredients:

- oz. (226.79 grams) of organic tuna steak, seared
- 1 pint of fresh cherry tomatoes
- 2-3 tablespoons of whole Niçoise olives, pitted
- 1 whole medium potato (boiled and pan sautéed in coconut oil)
- 1-2 eggs, poached
- 2 cups of spinach
- 4-6 filets of anchovies
- 8-10 leaves of butter lettuce
- 2-3 teaspoons of caper berries
- A pinch (or 2) of garlic powder
- Coconut oil, for cooking

For dressing:

- 3 tablespoons of Dijon mustard
- 1/2 tablespoon of organic olive oil
- Sea salt, to taste
- 1 tablespoon of coconut vinegar
- Black pepper, to taste

Method of preparation:

1.Boil the whole potatoes until slightly soft. Cut the boiled potatoes into slices and then sauté those in the coconut oil until crisp and set aside.

2.Add the spinach and stir-fry in using the same coconut oil mixed with garlic powder, add more oil if needed.

3.Add the tuna steaks and stir-fry so that they absorb coconut oil taste. Turn off the heat and set aside and let it cool down. The spinach will have an incredible taste!

4.To arrange the salad, lay the lettuce leaves flat on a salad platter and then arrange the eggs sunny side up. Arrange the rest of the salad as desired.

5.Finally, whisk all the ingredients of the dressing and drizzle over salad before serving. Enjoy!

Tuna with Roasted Broccoli Salad

Servings: 1-2
Preparation time: 20 minutes
Cooking time: 30-35 minutes

Ingredients:

- 2-3 cups of roasted broccoli, chopped into florets
- 6-8 pieces of whole green olives
- 5 oz. (141.7 grams) of wild caught tuna, drained
- 1/2 of a whole avocado, peeled and mashed
- 5 fresh cherry tomatoes, quartered
- 1/3 cup of almonds
- A pinch of sea salt
- 1 tablespoon of paleo Dijon mustard
- 1 tablespoon of olive oil
- 1-2 oz. of paleo feta cheese, diced (Optional)
- Black pepper, to taste

Method of preparation:

1.Chop the broccoli into florets and transfer to a baking dish. Drizzle over some olive oil.
2.Add the dried garlic, salt and black pepper to the broccoli florets.
3.Toss the broccoli florets with the added ingredients and transfer to a 400 degrees Fahrenheit preheated oven. Roast for 30-35 minutes.
4.Mix the tuna with the Dijon mustard, a pinch of sea salt and mashed avocado. Set aside.
5.Sauté the broccoli florets in some oil until crisp. Add the paleo vegan cheese to the pan and allow it to melt in the pan over the broccoli florets.
6.Set aside to cool down.
7.Toss the tuna with the broccoli florets and then add a little bit of olive oil, the almonds and the quartered cherry tomatoes to the mixture.
8.Toss the mixture to prepare the salad. Serve chilled. Enjoy!

Lemon Salmon Salad

Servings: 1-2

Preparation time: 5-8 minutes

Ingredients:

- 1 piece of cooked salmon darne, roughly chopped
- Flaked almonds
- 3.5oz. (100g) of spinach
- 6 pieces of sun-dried tomatoes, finely diced
- Juice from 1/4th lemon
- 2 tablespoons of powdered nuts
- 2 tablespoons of sliced scallions

Method of preparation:

1.Cut salmon darne pieces into bite sized pieces.

2.Toss all the other ingredients with the salmon and serve.

3.You can use your dinner leftovers and conjure up and incredibly healthy and energizing Paleo friendly salad for lunch or even for breakfast! Full-on energy!

Chopped Salad with Tuna

Servings: 2-3
Preparation time: 15 minutes
Cooking time: 5 minutes

Ingredients:

- 6-oz. (170 grams) of fresh water-packed tuna, wild caught and drained
- 1 celery stalk, chopped
- ½ cup of chopped radishes
- 1 whole cucumber,chopped
- 1 cup of chopped romaine lettuce
- 1 medium sized tomato, chopped
- 1 whole avocado, peeled, pitted and diced
- 1 carrot, chopped
- For the Dressing:
- 2 garlic cloves, minced
- 3 teaspoons of olive oil
- A pinch of Himalaya salt
- 2 tablespoons of fresh lime juice
- ½ teaspoon of ground black pepper

Method of preparation:

1.Place all the veggies in a salad bowl, cover and set aside.

2.Combine the dressing ingredients in another bowl. Finally, combine tuna with the salad in the bowl and toss lightly to mix.

3.Then drizzle the salad dressing over the vegetables and tuna salad and serve right away. Enjoy!

Avocado Codfish Salad

Servings: 5-6
Preparation time: 15-20 minutes
Cooking time: 1 hour

Ingredients:

- 1 Packet of organic salted codfish, boneless
- 1 whole avocado, pitted and diced
- 1 tomato, peeled, halved and sliced
- 1/2 teaspoon of adobo sauce (some experts say it's not really Paleo, so let's make it optional, unless you don't mind minor cheatings here and there)
- 1 red onion, peeled and chopped
- 2 fresh limes, juiced
- 2 teaspoons of olive oil
- Jalapeno
- 1 teaspoon of black pepper
- 1 teaspoon kosher salt
- A handful of chopped cilantro

Method of preparation:

1.Bring a pot of fresh water to boil and drop the cod fish in it.

2.Boil the fish for half an hour until soft. Once done, drain the water, remove the fish from heat and allow it to cool down. Once the fish cools down, cut it into bite sized squares.

3.Next chop the avocado, cilantro, onion and tomato to get medium sized pieces of vegetables.

4.Place the vegetables in a salad bowl. Add the cod fish pieces to the mixture.

5.Drizzle fresh juice of 2 limes, olive oil and adobo sauce over the salad. Season with kosher salt and black pepper as required and toss the salad to blend the flavors. Serve immediately.

Escondido Codfish Salad

Servings: 4
Preparation time: 1 hour 15 minutes
Cooking time: 5-7 minutes

Ingredients:
- 1 lb. (453.6 grams) fillet of fresh codfish
- 1 large green bell pepper (seeded and diced
- ½ lb. (226.8 grams) of jicama (peeled and grated)
- ½ cup of fresh lime juice
- 1 small sized jalapeno chili (seeded and minced)
- ½ cup of fresh lemon juice
- 2 scallions, minced
- 2 tablespoons of paleo coconut vinegar
- 1 tablespoon of lime rind (grated)
- ½ cup of mint leaves
- ½ cup of basil leaves
- 4 tablespoons of olive oil
- 2 whole carrots, peeled, grated
- ½ teaspoon of salt, plus more to taste
- 1 cup of coriander leaves
- 1 teaspoon ground pepper

Method of preparation:
1. Bring a pot full of 1 inch up water to boil.
2. Place a slotted tray over the pot and put the cod fish fillet over the plate.
3. Steam the fish for 5-7 minutes.
4. Once done, cool down the fish in the refrigerator. Once chilled, remove from the refrigerator and shred the fish. Set aside.
5. In a bowl, whisk the lemon juice, sugar, lime rind, jalapeno, salt and lime juice. Add in the olive oil after whisking the lemon juice mixture for a few seconds.
6. Dip the shredded cod fish in the lemon juice mixture and toss. Place back in refrigerator and let refrigerate for 1 hour.
7. Remove from fridge after 1 hour and add all the other remaining ingredients. Toss well and serve!

Smoked Mackerel and New Potato Salad

Servings: 2
Preparation time: 15 minutes
Cooking time: 15- 20 minutes

Ingredients:

- 7 oz. (200 grams) of smoked mackerel fillets, skinned and flaked
- 12 oz. (350 grams) of new potatoes
- 1 teaspoon of horseradish cream
- 3.5 oz. (100 grams) of coconut yoghurt
- 3 oz. (85 grams) of fresh watercress
- Juice of 1 lemon
- A dash of ground black pepper

Method of preparation:

1.Rinse the potatoes very nicely under running water, as new potatoes tend to have a lot of dirt on them. Rinse the potatoes until the water turns clear and no longer retains the murkiness. Bring a pot of salted water to boil and once the water starts boiling, drop the rinsed new potatoes in the pot. Let the potatoes boil in the water until tender, which will take approximately 15-20 minutes.

2.While the potatoes are boiling, mix up the coconut yoghurt, horseradish cream and fresh lemon juice in a big bowl.

3.Season with some black pepper and stir slightly to combine well and to get a lump free smooth dressing.

4.Once the potatoes are cooked, drain them off and cool them down.

5.Then cut them in halves. Leave aside.

6.Add the smoked mackerel and the watercress to the yoghurt dressing and toss. Finally add the halved potatoes and toss again to coat. Serve the warm salad right away.

Khmer Fish Salad

Servings: 2
Preparation time: 10 minutes

Ingredients:

- 3oz. (80 grams) of snapper fillet, finely sliced
- A bunch of asparagus, chopped and previously boiled
- 0.881 oz. (25 grams) of white cabbage, thinly sliced
- A handful of fresh mint leaves
- 0.881 oz. (25 grams) of purple cabbage, thinly sliced
- 2 fresh red Asian shallots, thinly sliced
- 0.881 oz. (25 grams) of iceberg lettuce, thinly sliced
- A handful of fresh spinach
- 2 teaspoon of organic raw honey
- 1 Lebanese cucumber, julienned
- 3oz. (80 grams) of green capsicum, thinly sliced
- 1 teaspoon of paleo fish sauce
- A handful of fresh Vietnamese mint leaves
- 1 whole carrot, julienned
- A handful of fresh Thai basil leaves

For the lime marinade:

- 0.405 fl. oz. (12 ml) of fresh lime juice
- A pinch of thinly sliced lemongrass, white part only
- 1 teaspoon of coriander paste
- A pinch of sea salt
- Garnish:
- Sliced red chilies
- Roasted unsalted crushed peanuts

Method of preparation:

Slice up all the vegetables (carrot, iceberg lettuce, asparagus, cucumber, purple cabbage, green capsicum, white cabbage and Asian shallots) and dump in a large salad bowl.

Now slice the snapper fillet in diagonal sections across the bone and place in a bowl. Add 12 ml of fresh lime juice, coriander paste and thinly sliced lemongrass to the fish slices and give a gentle toss to the mixture.

Let the fish marinate in the marinade for 10-12 minutes or until the fish turns its color into opaque white. Once done, strain the fish slices from the marinade and squeeze out all of the marinade from the fish slices. Set the fish slices aside to be used later. Add the spinach and fresh herbs and mix well with the veggies. Now combine the fish slices to the salad and add the fish sauce, honey and the reserved lime marinade to the salad. Toss the entire salad gently a few times and serve straight away.

<u>Warm Fish Salad</u>

Servings: 4
Preparation time: 20 minutes
Cooking time: 6-8 minutes

Ingredients:

* 24.69 oz. (700 grams) of white fish fillets, skinless
* 1 medium sized Lebanese cucumber, thinly sliced
* oz. (120 grams) of Asian salad mix
* 1 small sized red capsicum, (remove the seeds and slice)
* 1-2 tablespoons of olive oil, to coat
* 1½ cups of fresh spinach
* 1 small sized carrot, julienned
* For the dressing:
* 2 tablespoons of raw organic honey
* Fresh juice of 1 lemon
* 2 cloves of garlic, thinly chopped
* 1½ tablespoons of paleo fish sauce
* 1 teaspoon of fresh grated ginger
* 1 teaspoon of sesame oil
* 1 small sized red chili, chopped

Method of preparation:

1. Heat up a charcoal grill to moderate heat.
2. Then, slice the fish filets into bite sized (3-4 cm) pieces and dump in a bowl. Drizzle vegetable oil over the fish pieces and toss the pieces to coat those nicely on all sides with the oil.
3. Take a saucepan of hot water and drop the spinach leaves. Blanch for a few minutes and then strain immediately to avoid overcooking.
4. Combine in a bowl all of the dressing ingredients and set aside.
5. Now place the fish slices on the hot prepared grill and grill for approximately 2-3 minutes on each side of the fish or until the fish slices turn tender and develop light grill marks on them.
6. Once done, let the grilled fish cool down a bit and then mix it with the veggies and the dressing. Enjoy!

Grilled Fish and Zucchini Salad

Servings: 2
Preparation time: 10 minutes
Cooking time: 30 minutes

Ingredients:

- 2 big zucchini, cut into chunks
- 2 white fish filets
- Olive oil, (1 teaspoon)
- 3 oz. (85 grams) of roasted red peppers, chopped
- 6 pitted black olives
- A bunch of fresh rocket leaves
- 1 large clove of garlic, crushed
- 1 tablespoon of paleo mayonnaise
- A pinch of sea salt
- Ground black, freshly crushed

Method of preparation:

1. Heat up a grill and place a heavy duty foil over the grill. Grease it with some oil.

2. Now take the fish filets and grease those with oil as well. Season the fish filets with salt and pepper and let then place the filets over the hot grill.

3. Let the fish filets sit on the grill for 6-8 minutes or until the fish is cooked all the way through and starts to flake pretty easily.

4. Boil the zucchini (low heat) for 15 minutes until soft. Avoid overcooking. Once done, drain the water from the pot and dump the potatoes in a pan.

5. Stir the olives, crushed garlic and roasted red peppers with the boiled potatoes in the pan. Finally, add-in the paleo mayonnaise and stir lightly to combine.

6. Serve the grilled fish pieces salad over the rocket leaves and the zucchini mixture.

Easy Tuna and Spinach Salad

Servings: 4-6
Preparation time: 15 minutes

Ingredients:

- 14 oz. (400 grams) of wild caught fresh tuna fish in oil
- 2 oz. (56.7 grams) red onion, sliced
- 9 oz. (250 g) of radish
- 1 oz. (25 grams) of fresh rocket leaves

For the dressing:

- 2 cloves of garlic, peeled
- 3 tablespoons of fresh lemon juice
- 1 teaspoon mustard powder
- 2 tablespoons of olive oil
- A pinch of salt
- Zest of 1 big lemon
- 1 teaspoon of black peppercorns

Method of preparation:

1.Drain the tuna fish from the oil and reserve the oil. Set aside both the fish pieces and the oil for later use.
2.Press the garlic cloves with sea salt in a mortar and pestle and then add the mustard powder to the mixture. Process again to combine.
3.Grind the peppercorns in as well and then add the lemon juice, 3 tablespoons of reserved tuna oil, zest of lemon and extra virgin olive oil to the garlic mixture in the mortar. Mix everything up nicely with a spoon to prepare the salad dressing and then keep aside.
4.Coat the rocket leaves with the dressing, make sure all the leaves are nicely covered for optimal taste. Add the rest of the ingredients and top with tuna chunks. Serve immediately, enjoy!

Fish Fillets with Cress and Avocado Salad

Servings: 1
Preparation time: 10-15 minutes
Cooking time: 7-8 minutes

Ingredients:
- 6 oz. (170 grams) of white fish fillets, skin removed
- A bunch of watercress
- 1 egg, nicely beaten
- 2 tablespoons of almond flour
- Juice of 1/2 a lemon
- 1/2 of a red chili, deseeded and chopped finely
- 2 oz. (56.7 grams) of almond powder
- 1 whole ripe avocado (peeled, pitted and sliced)
- 1 tablespoon olive oil
- Sea salt
- A pinch of black pepper

Method of preparation:

1.Prepare a frying pan by putting some oil in it. Place the pan on medium high heat.
2.While the pan is getting ready, mix up the almond flour with ground black pepper and sea salt.
3.Beat the egg in another bowl and keep the bowl aside.
4.Take the fish filets and dump those one by one in the almond flour mixture. Coat with the mixture of flour nicely on all sides and thereafter, transfer the filets immediately to the bowl of the beaten eggs.
5.Dip the fish filets in the egg and then coat with some almond powder. Once done, fry the "paleo cheese"coated fish filets in the heated pan after greasing that with a little bit of oil. Let the filets brown a bit while frying. Add the red chili after a few minutes and stir fry for a few seconds.
6.Toss the watercress and avocado with lemon juice and some olive oil.

7.Put all of these ingredients in a plate and top with the fish filets to serve.

Section 3

Chicken Paleo Salads

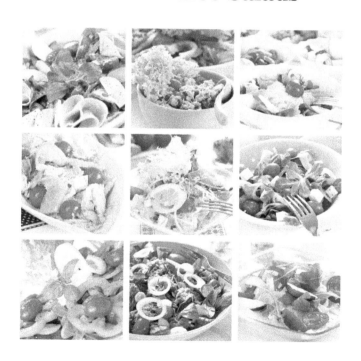

Pink Chicken Salad

Servings: 4

Preparation time: 1 hour

Ingredients:

- 1½ lbs. (680.3 grams) of cooked chicken, shredded
- 3/4 cup of dried cranberries
- 3/4 cup of diced celery
- 2 teaspoons of sea salt
- 2 fresh green onions, diced
- ½ cup of fresh grapes, sliced in half
- 1½ teaspoons of black pepper
- ¾ cup of strained coconut yogurt
- 1 teaspoon of smoked paprika

Method of preparation:

1. Dice and chop the vegetables as required. Transfer all of those to a salad bowl.

2. Mix all the other ingredients and then toss all to combine.

3. Transfer to refrigerator and let chill for 1 hour or more before serving.

4. Serve over home-made paleo gluten free bread or lettuce leaves.

Avocado Chicken Salad

Servings: 2-3

Preparation time: 5 minutes

Ingredients:

- 1 lb. (453.592 grams) chicken, cooked and shredded

- 4 tablespoons of onions, finely diced

- 3 whole avocados

- Black pepper

- 1 medium sized fresh tomato, diced

- A pinch of sea salt

- 4 whole limes, juiced

Method of preparation:

1.Peel and pit the avocados and mash those. Add all the other ingredients.

2.Combine the added ingredients with the avocado and serve. Enjoy!

Curry Love Chicken Salad

Servings: 6
Preparation time: 10 minutes
Cooking time: 10 minutes

Ingredients:

- 12 oz. (340 grams) of chicken (cooked and diced)
- 6 radicchio cups
- 1 cup of walnut halves
- 1/2 cup of mayonnaise
- 1 cup of red grapes
- 2 tablespoons of coconut vinegar
- 1 large celery rib, halved lengthwise and thinly sliced crosswise
- 2 scallions, trimmed and thinly sliced
- 1/3 cup of coconut vinegar
- 3 oz. (85 grams) of mixed baby greens
- ¼ teaspoon of curry powder
- ¼ teaspoon of black pepper

Method of preparation:

1.Toast the walnuts in a 375 degrees Fahrenheit oven for 10 minutes. Chop coarsely after done.

2.Toss 3/4th of the walnuts with chicken, celery and grapes in a salad bowl.

3.In another bowl, mix the paleo mayonnaise, scallions, curry powder, coconut vinegar and black pepper.

4.Cover the chicken and walnuts with the dressing and toss well.

5.Serve in radicchio cups and sprinkle the greens around it.

Grilled Chicken Salad with Mango and Avocado

Servings: 4
Preparation time: 15 minutes
Cooking time: 8 minutes

Ingredients:

- 4 skinless chicken breast halves (remove the bones)
- 2 tablespoons of mango chutney
- cups of mixed salad greens
- 2 tablespoons of olive oil
- 1 cup of peeled and diced mango
- 2 tablespoons of fresh lime juice
- 3/4th cup of avocado, peeled and diced
- 1 tablespoon of coconut aminos
- Cooking spray
- 3/4th teaspoon of grated fresh ginger

Method of preparation:

1. Preheat a grill and grease it with some cooking spray.
2. Take a bowl and combine the coconut aminos, chutney, lime juice, olive oil and ginger in it. Keep aside.
3. Lay the chicken breast halves on a flat surface and brush those with 2 tablespoons of the chutney mixture.
4. Grill the chicken for 4 minutes on each side while coating lightly with the chutney mixture again on flipping. Remove from grill once done.
5. Cut the chicken into diagonal pieces. Lay the avocado slices, mango slices and salad greens on the plate and place the chicken pieces on top to serve. Enjoy!

Holiday Chicken Salad

Servings: 12

Preparation time: 15 minutes

Cooking time: 15 minutes

Ingredients:

* 4 cups of cooked chicken, cubed
* 1 cup of celery, chopped
* 1 cup of chopped pecans
* Half cup of paleo mayonnaise (preferably homemade)
* Sea salt, to taste
* 1/2 cup of minced green bell pepper
* 1 1/2 cups of dried cranberries (organic and paleo)
* 1 teaspoon paleo seasoning salt
* 2 fresh green onions, chopped
* 1 teaspoon of paprika
* Ground black pepper, to taste

Method of preparation:

1.Combine the Paleo mayonnaise with seasoning salt and paprika.

2.Add all the veggies and fruits. Then, combine the chicken pieces with the mixture at the last.

3.Insert the salad in refrigerator and let chill for 1-2 hours before serving.

4.Serve in lettuce leaves cups or in bell pepper cups or over paleo breads.

<u>Creamy Chicken Salad</u>

Servings: 6
Preparation time: 2 hours
Cooking time: 40-45 minutes

Ingredients:

- 2 lbs. (907 grams) of skinless chicken breasts (no bones), halved
- 1 tablespoon of lime juice
- 1 tablespoon of Dijon mustard
- 1/2 cup of light paleo mayonnaise
- 1/2 cup Greek style coconut yogurt
- 1/3 cup of celery, chopped
- 1 tablespoon of paleo coconut vinegar
- 1/3 cup of paleo unsweetened dried cranberries (organic)
- 1 teaspoon of pure raw honey
- 2 oz. (56.699 grams) of smoked almonds
- 1/2 teaspoon of kosher salt
- 6 cups of mixed salad greens
- A pinch of black pepper

Method of preparation:

1.Fill up a Dutch oven two thirds up with water. Bring the water to boil.

2.Wrap up each piece of chicken breast halves with heavy duty plastic wraps and drop in the boiling water.

3.Lower the heat a bit.

4.Let the chicken simmer for 40-45 minutes. Once done, unwrap the chicken breast pieces and shred those. Let cool and transfer to refrigerator to allow chilling for 30-40 minutes.

5.Mix the mayonnaise with shredded chicken, cranberries, celery, almonds and the rest. Chill the salad for 1 hour. Enjoy!

Mediterranean Chicken Salad

Servings: 3-4

Preparation time: 10 minutes

Ingredients:

- 1 lb. (458 grams) of roasted chicken (organic and paleo)

- 1 head of butter or romaine lettuce

- 1/2 cup of paleo mayonnaise (preferably homemade)

- 1 whole lemon, juiced

- 4 tablespoons of fresh cilantro, roughly chopped

- 1 whole red onion, diced

- Sea salt

- Black pepper

Method of preparation:

1.Shred the roasted chicken mix it well with rest of the ingredients, except the lettuce leaves.

2.Serve the salad as it is or chilled in the lettuce "boats".

Chicken Larb Recipe

Servings: 4
Preparation time: 10 minutes
Cooking time: 10-12 minutes

Ingredients:

- 1 1/2 lbs. (680.388 grams) of ground chicken
- 3/4 cup of homemade chicken stock (paleo)
- 2/3 cup of fresh lime juice
- 2 tablespoons of lemongrass (minced or powdered)
- 1/3 cup of mint leaves
- 1/3 cup of paleo fish sauce
- A few chopped cilantro leaves
- 1 tablespoon of raw paleo honey
- 2 teaspoons of paleo chili-garlic sauce
- Kosher salt, to taste
- 1 cup of green onions, sliced
- 3/4 cup shallots, sliced
- 1 whole head of fresh butter lettuce
- 1 tablespoon of Serrano chili, thinly sliced

Method of preparation:

1.Heat up the chicken stock in a stock pot and drop the ground chicken in it. Simmer the chicken for 6-8 minutes while stirring it occasionally to break the lumps. Add the shallots, lemongrass, green onions and Serrano chilies.

2.In the meantime, combine the honey, fish sauce, lime juice and chili garlic sauce in a bowl and set aside (our salad dressing)
Stir and cook the chicken for 4-5 minutes or until the shallots turn translucent.

3.Once cooked, drain the entire liquid from the stock pot and then toss the chicken mixture with the chili garlic sauce mixture.
Serve in lettuce leaves boats.

Chipotle Chicken Salad

Servings: 2-3

Preparation time: 10 minutes

Ingredients:

- 1 lb. (453.592 grams) of cooked chicken, diced
- 1/4 of a white onion (peeled, chopped)
- 4 stalks of celery, finely chopped

For the Paleo mayonnaise (non-vegan):

- 2/3 cup of organic avocado oil
- A pinch of black pepper
- 1 organic egg
- Sea salt
- Fresh lemon juice (1 teaspoon)
- 1/4 teaspoon of organic garlic powder
- 1 teaspoon chipotle adobo sauce (paleo)
- Black pepper, to taste

Method of preparation:

1.To prepare the mayonnaise, blend all the mayonnaise ingredients in a bowl until completely blended and smooth.

2.Mix the chicken with celery and white onions. Add some Paleo mayo and serve. Enjoy!

<u>Classic Chicken Salad</u>

Servings: 5-6

Preparation time: 10 minutes

Ingredients:

- 2 lbs. (907 grams) of cooked chicken, cubed or shredded
- 2-3 stalks celery, chopped
- 1 cup of fresh grapes, cut in halves
- 1/3 cup of pecans, chopped (optional)
- 1/2 cup of apple, peeled and chopped (optional)
- 5 teaspoons lemon garlic pepper (paleo)
- 1/2 cup of chopped white or red onion
- 1 cup of paleo mayo (check out the previous recipes)
- 1/2-1 tablespoon of fresh lemon juice
- 2 teaspoons of paleo Trader Joe's 21 Seasoning Salute
- 1 teaspoon of sea salt

Method of preparation:

1.Cube or shred the chicken and add all the fruits, vegetables and nuts to the chicken after chopping and cutting those in the manner as is mentioned.

2.Slowly add the mayonnaise and then add the seasoning, sea salt and pepper. Give a light toss to the salad and serve right away.

Chicken with Roasted Asparagus and Bacon Salad

Servings: 2
Preparation time: 10-15 minutes
Cooking time: 10-15 minutes

Ingredients:
- 4 slices of thick cut bacon, paleo
- 6 oz. (200g) of leftover cooked chicken, cut into bite size pieces
- 1 whole ripe avocado, peeled pitted and sliced
- 1/2 cup of asparagus, chopped into 2-3 inch pieces
- 4 cups of baby spinach leaves, chopped
- For the vinaigrette:
- A few tablespoons of olive oil
- 1 teaspoon Dijon mustard
- 2 tablespoons of paleo balsamic vinegar
- 2 teaspoons rosemary, finely chopped
- 1 large clove garlic (peeled and minced)
- 1 tablespoon of thyme, minced
- 1/2 teaspoon of black pepper
- A pinch of Himalayan salt

Method of preparation:

1.Cook the bacon over medium heat in a pan until the bacon slices turn brown and crispy. Once that happens, drain the bacon slices from the pan using a slotted spoon and set aside.

2.Chop the asparagus and dump in the same pan over the bacon drippings. Stir fry the asparagus for 4-5 minutes or until the asparagus gets imbued with the bacon flavors. Turn off the heat once done and set the pan aside.

3.Now dump all the ingredients for the vinaigrette in a small bowl or glass jar and whisk with a metal whisk to get the vinaigrette. The vinaigrette should have a bit emulsified look.

4.Lay the baby spinach leaves over a salad platter and sprinkle the cooked chicken pieces and bacon bits over the spinach. Add the

156

avocado slices as well and then drizzle a little bit of vinaigrette on top to serve immediately.

Kiwi-Strawberry Chicken Tender Salad

Servings: 2
Preparation time: 30-40 minutes
Cooking time: 22 minutes

Ingredients:
- 1 lb. (453.592 grams) of chicken cutlets, cut vertically into tenders
- 1 cup of almond flour
- 1 organic egg
- 1½ whole kiwis
- 4 tablespoons of organic raisins
- 1/4th lb. (113 grams) of strawberries
- 3 oz. (85 grams) of fresh baby spinach
- 1 tablespoon of maple syrup, organic and paleo
- 1 whole fresh avocado
- 5 strawberries, sliced
- Sea salt, to taste
- 2 teaspoons of organic honey
- Black pepper, to taste
- Juice of ½ organic lemon
- 1 cup of shredded carrots
- Cucumber, sliced

Method of preparation:

1.Process the 1/4th lb. of strawberries and kiwis in a juicer to extract the juice of these fruits. Mix and combine the maple syrup thoroughly with the strawberry kiwi juice and set aside.

2.Whisk the egg in another bowl and add 2 tablespoons worth of the strawberry kiwi juice and a dash of sea salt and black pepper to it. Stir to combine.

3.Take the almond flour in another separate bowl.
Slice up the chicken cutlets into thin chicken tenders. Take a chicken tender and dunk that in the egg mixture. Transfer the chicken tenders

to the almond flour and coat nicely on all sides. Once done, transfer the coated chicken tenders to a greased baking sheet. Repeat the same process with all the remaining chicken tenders.

4.Bake the chicken tenders in a 400 degrees Fahrenheit preheated oven for 20 minutes. Then turn on the broil and broil those for an additional 2 minutes.

5.In the meantime, prepare the salad while the chicken is baking. For that, place half of the fresh baby spinach leaves in a bowl. Dump the avocado in the bowl and add 2 tablespoons worth of the strawberry kiwi juice to the avocado. Mash the avocado with the juices into the spinach.

6.Then add the shredded carrots, 4 sliced strawberries, raisins, lemon juice and a dash of salt and pepper to the salad.

7.Then add the remaining strawberry and cucumbers. Finally top with the baked chicken tenders.

8.Mix the remaining honey with the strawberry kiwi juice and drizzle that over the salad. Enjoy!

Shawarma Chicken Salad with Basil-Lemon Vinaigrette

Servings: 4
Preparation time: 10 minutes
Cooking time: 13 hours

Ingredients for shawarma:

- 1 lb. (453 grams) of free-range chicken breasts, sliced into 3-inch sized strips
- 3 minced garlic cloves,
- 1 tablespoon of olive oil
- A pinch of ground cumin
- 2 tablespoons of fresh lemon juice
- 1 teaspoon curry powder
- ¾ teaspoon of fine grain sea salt
- ¼ teaspoon of ground coriander

Salad:

- oz. (100 grams) of fresh spring greens
- 2 handfuls of fresh basil leaves, torn roughly
- 5oz. (150 grams) of fresh cherry tomatoes cut in halves
- 1 whole avocado, peeled, pitted and sliced

Basil-Lemon Vinaigrette:

- 1 clove of garlic, peeled and smashed
- 2 large handfuls of fresh basil leaves
- 5 tablespoons olive oil
- ½ teaspoon of fine grained sea salt
- 2 tablespoons of lemon juice

Method of preparation:

1.Whisk lemon juice, olive oil, curry powder, cumin, garlic, coriander and salt in a bowl to prepare the marinade.

2.Pack the chicken strips into a sealable pouch and add the marinade. Seal and let the chicken sit in the marinade overnight or at least for 20 minutes.

3.When ready to cook, take a skillet and heat up a little amount of olive oil and fry the marinated chicken over medium heat, until the chicken strips attain a golden brown color, for about 6-8 minutes.

4.To prepare the vinaigrette, process the basil, lemon juice, garlic and sea salt in a food processor.

5.Once the mixture turns pasty, start adding the olive oil slowly. Process for a couple of minutes, until you obtain well-combined and smooth vinaigrette.

6.In a bowl, toss the salad green with some salt and pepper and drop the cherry tomatoes, avocado slices, basil and cooked chicken pieces on top. Finally, drizzle the vinaigrette on top and serve. Enjoy!

Chicken Salad with Spinach and Strawberries

Servings: 2 - 4
Preparation time: 15-20 minutes

Ingredients:

- 12 oz. (340 grams) of cooked chicken, cubed
- 2 cups of fresh strawberries, sliced
- oz. (227 grams) of fresh baby spinach
- 4 tablespoons of chopped walnuts

Dressing:

- 1 tablespoon of coconut vinegar
- 4 tablespoons of walnut oil
- 1/2 teaspoon of paleo Dijon mustard
- 1 teaspoon of raw honey
- Some pepper
- Sea salt, to taste

Method of preparation:

1.Whisk the honey, walnut oil, Dijon mustard, coconut vinegar, ground black pepper and sea salt in a bowl until the dressing becomes smooth and you get a well combined dressing.

2.Slice the strawberries, chop the walnuts and cut the chicken into small cubes.

3.Combine the spinach with walnuts, strawberries and chicken and drizzle the prepared dressing over the salad.

4.Toss the salad lightly to mix well and serve immediately. Enjoy!

Chicken with Charred Tomato and Broccoli Salad

Servings: 6
Preparation time: 20-25 minutes
Cooking time: 10-15 minutes

Ingredients:

* 3 cups of cooked chicken breast, shredded
* 1 1/2 lbs. (680 grams) of medium sized ripe tomatoes
* 1/4th cup of fresh lemon juice
* 3 tablespoons of olive oil
* 4 cups broccoli florets
* A pinch (or more if you like it hot) of chili powder
* 2 teaspoons of extra-virgin olive oil
* 1 teaspoon of sea salt
* Crackled black pepper (1 teaspoon)

Method of preparation:

1.Boil the broccoli florets in a pot of boiling water for about 3-5 minutes Once they get soft, drain the broccoli florets and place the hot florets under some running cold water until the florets cool down.

2.Cut the tomatoes in half horizontally and let the juices and seeds run out. In the meantime, heat up a skillet over high heat. Brush the tops of the halved tomatoes with oil and place those cut side down in the hot pan and let cook for 4-5 minutes or until the tomatoes soften up.

3.Brush the tomatoes again with a teaspoon of olive oil and place back in the pan to let the skin get charred for 1-2 minutes. Once done, remove the tomatoes from the pan.

4.Add some olive oil to the pan and add sea salt, chili powder and ground black pepper. Stir the mixture constantly and cook for 40-45 minutes or until the mixture turns fragrant. Then add in the lemon juice, stir well to combine and then remove from heat.

163

5.Chop the tomatoes and then toss the tomatoes with shredded chicken and broccoli florets. Drizzle some lemon juice dressing, serve and enjoy!

Chicken Salad with Pecans and Cherries

Servings: 4
Preparation time: 20-30 minutes
Cooking time: 20-25 minutes

Ingredients:

- 1 1/4 lbs. (567 grams) of chicken breasts, skinless and boneless trimmed
- 1/3 cup of paleo mayonnaise
- 1/2 cup of celery (sliced)
- 1/2 cup of pecans, slightly toasted and chopped
- 1 head of butterhead lettuce, chopped
- 1/2 cup of dried cherries
- 1/3 cup of coconut yogurt
- A pinch of sea salt
- 1 tablespoon raw honey mustard

Method of preparation:

1.Fill up a pot with some water and add 1/4th teaspoon of sea salt to it. Bring the water in the pot to boil and then drop the chicken breasts in it. Once the chicken breasts start boiling, reduce the heat and cover the pot with a lid. Let the chicken simmer for 20-25 minutes or until the time those are cooked through, tender and are no longer pink. Once done, drain the water and let the chicken cool down.

2.Mix up the paleo mayonnaise with coconut yoghurt, black pepper, mustard and remaining salt in a bowl.

3.Cut up the chicken breasts into small pieces once the chicken breasts cool down.

4.Toss the chicken pieces with cherries, celery and pecans. Add the prepared mayonnaise dressing and mix well.

5.Serve the salad over the lettuce. Enjoy!

Chopped Chicken Greek Salad

Servings: 4
Preparation time: 15-20 minutes

Ingredients:

- 12 oz. (340 grams) of cooked chicken, chopped
- 6 cups of chopped romaine lettuce
- 1/2 cup of crumbled paleo feta cheese***
- Optional: 1/3 cup of paleo vinegar (or red wine- allowed on Paleo)
- 2 medium sized tomatoes, chopped
- 2 tablespoons of olive oil (extra-virgin)
- 1/2 cup of sliced ripe black olives
- 1 tablespoon of fresh dill, chopped
- 1 medium sized cucumber, peeled, chopped
- 1 teaspoon of garlic powder
- 1/4 teaspoon Himalaya salt
- 1 onion, chopped
- A pinch of freshly ground pepper

***To make Paleo Cashew Feta Style Cheese, simply blend the following ingredients: 1 cup of raw cashews previously soaked in water for at least a few hours (I leave it to soak overnight and I use alkaline water), about ¼ cup of almond milk or coconut milk, 1 tablespoon of lime juice, ¼ cup of nutritional yeast, 1 clove of garlic and a bit of Himalaya salt to taste. Transfer into little cubes (like for ice making) and store in a fridge for a few hours.

Method of preparation:

1.Toss the olives, romaine lettuce, paleo feta cheese, cucumber, onions, tomatoes and chicken cubes in a bowl.
2.Whisk some olive oil, red wine, dill, ground black pepper and sea salt in a bowl.
3.Drizzle the dressing over the salad and toss again before serving.
4.Enjoy!

Orange Five Spice Chicken Salad

Servings: 4
Preparation time: 15-20 minutes
Cooking time: 15-17 minutes

Ingredients:

- 1 lb. (458 grams) of skinless and boneless chicken breasts, trimmed
- 3 whole fresh oranges
- 1 tablespoon of Dijon mustard
- 12 cups of mixed Asian greens
- 3 tablespoons of coconut vinegar
- 6 teaspoons of extra-virgin olive oil
- 1 red bell pepper, with no seeds
- 1 teaspoon of five-spice powder, organic
- 1/2 cup of slivered red onion
- 1 teaspoon of kosher salt, divided
- A pinch of freshly ground black pepper

Method of preparation:

1.In a bowl, combine the five spice powder, some olive oil, salt and black pepper so as to prepare a spice rub.

2. the chicken breast pieces with the spice rub.

3.In a skillet, heat up a bit of olive oil and brown the spiced chicken pieces. Once browned on one side, flip the chicken pieces and pop the skillet into a 450 degrees Fahrenheit oven.

4.Roast the chicken in the oven for about 10 minutes.

5.Once cooked, set aside to cool down.

6.Finally, shred the chicken and toss with the salad ingredients. Enjoy!

Section 4

More Amazing Paleo Salads

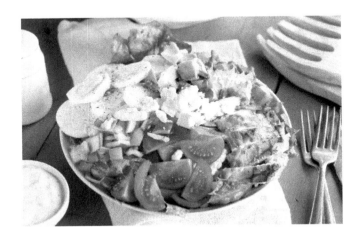

Red Potato Honey Mustard Salad

Servings: 4
Preparation time: 15 minutes
Cooking time: 15 minutes

Ingredients:

- 3 lbs. (1.36 kg) of red potatoes, cut into 1inch sized pieces
- 3 slices of thick cut bacon
- 3 tablespoons of homemade paleo mayonnaise
- 3 tablespoons of organic honey
- 2 medium sized onions, peeled and chopped
- 4 tablespoons of Dijon mustard
- 3 tablespoons of organic coconut vinegar
- 1/3rd cup of parsley
- 1 teaspoon of black pepper
- ½ teaspoon of sea salt

Method of preparation:

1.Boil the red potatoes in a pot of water and once boiling, lower the heat to simmer until the potatoes are cooked through and can be pierced with a knife or fork. Drain and set aside.
2.In the meantime, cook the bacon slices until all the fat is released.
3.Add the onion slices and sauté those in bacon fat until caramelized.
4.Prepare the honey dressing by mixing mayonnaise, honey, Dijon mustard and coconut vinegar.
5.Toss the potatoes with sea salt, bacon and onion mixture, parsley and black pepper. Serve immediately or after chilling. Enjoy!

Duck with Sprout and Brussels Salad

Servings: 2
Preparation time: 15 minutes
Cooking time: 30-35 minutes

Ingredients:
- 2 pieces of duck breasts, skin on
- 2 whole clementine oranges
- 4 cups of Brussels sprouts, quartered
- 1/3 cup of organic dried cranberries
- 2 fennel stalks, finely chopped
- 1 tablespoon of coconut oil
- Coconut aminos (2 tablespoons)
- 2 teaspoons of black pepper
- 2 teaspoons of sea salt

Method of preparation:

1.Set up a temperature preheating of 375 degrees Fahrenheit on an oven. Scour the skin of duck breasts lightly on both sides and then sprinkle a dash of ground black pepper and sea salt on both the sides to season.

2.Transfer duck breasts to a skillet and cover the skillet with a parchment paper. Cook the duck for about 15 minutes and then flip.

3.Drain half of the coconut oil from skillet and transfer the skillet to the preheated oven.

4.Allow the duck to bake for 10-15 minutes.

5.While the duck is baking in the oven, heat up reserved coconut oil and fry the Brussels sprouts, cranberries and fennel in it. Stir and cook for a minute and then add the coconut aminos.

6. Stir to combine well. Then cook for 7-8 minutes or until the sprouts turn tender.

7.Slice the duck breasts and serve over cooked sprouts mixture. Drizzle clementine juice on top to serve.

Paleo Turkey Salad

Servings: 2

Preparation time: 10 minutes

Ingredients:

- 0.55 oz. (250g) of cooked turkey, cubed
- 4 tablespoons of chopped walnuts
- 1 whole avocado, peeled and diced
- 1/2 cup of fresh cranberries, halved
- 3 whole clementine oranges, sections halved
- 4 tablespoons of raw raisins
- 1 large endive, julienned
- 1/4 cup of fresh parsley
- 1/2 cup raw broccoli florets, chopped finely

Method of preparation:

1.Peel, cut and chop the vegetables and fruits as is required and mentioned in ingredients list.

2.Combine all of the added ingredients using a large salad bowl. Toss the salad and serve with dressing of choice or refrigerate for later use. Enjoy!

Paleo Taco Salad

Servings: 5-6

Preparation time: 15 minutes

Cooking time: 10 minutes

Ingredients:

- 2 lbs. (907 grams) of organic ground beef, cooked (leftovers will work well)
- 1 lb. (453.592 grams) of cooked bacon bits (organic)
- 1 large sized head of lettuce
- 3 whole avocados, peeled and pitted
- Paleo chimichurri (optional)
- Olive oil
- 2 whole fresh tomatoes
- 2 fresh red apples
- Apple cider vinegar (optional)
- Ground black pepper
- Sea salt

Method of preparation:

1.Season the meat with salt, olive oil and black pepper as required. Cool down if necessary.

2.Mix the cooled browned ground beef with the rest of the ingredients. Enjoy!

__Salade Lyonnaise__

Servings: 2

Preparations time: 15-20 minutes

Cooking time: 15-17 minutes

Ingredients:

- 1/4th lb. (113.398 grams) of thick-cut bacon

- 4 cups of fresh salad greens

- 2 poached eggs, organic

- 2 tablespoons of minced shallot

- 1 teaspoon of coconut vinegar

- Black pepper, to taste

- 1 tablespoon of organic ground mustard

- Salt, to taste

Method of preparation:

1.Bring a pot of water to boil and heat up another pan. Once water steams up, drop the eggs one by one at a time in it to poach those.

2.Fry the bacon bits for 10-12 minutes or unless those are browned and crispy. Season as required. Drain bacon bits in paper towels and set aside.

3.Cook the shallots lightly in the bacon fat and then add the mustard and vinegar. Stir nicely to mix. Then, cook for a couple of minutes.

4.Toss the salad greens with shallot mustard mixture and then serve with the bacon bits and pierced poached eggs on top. Enjoy!

Paleo Indonesian Shrimp Salad

Servings: 3-4
Preparation time: 10-15 minutes

Ingredients:

- 1 lb. (453.592 grams) of cooked shrimp, halved vertically
- 1.5 tablespoons of paleo fish sauce
- 3 whole fresh carrots, roughly shredded
- 6 tablespoons of raw almond butter (paleo)
- 1 whole seedless cucumber, julienned
- 6 tablespoons of raw unsweetened coconut milk (organic and paleo)
- 1 yellow or red bell pepper, seeded and sliced very thinly
- 1 teaspoon of paleo home-made sriracha sauce
- Raw organic cashews nuts, for garnishing
- 2 teaspoons of organic palm sugar (optional)
- 1 tablespoon of chopped scallions, for garnishing
- Juice of 1/2 lime
- 2 romaine lettuce hearts, coarsely shredded
- Lime wedges, for garnishing

Here's how to make your own sriracha sauce, all you need is a blender and:

- 1 cup of red jalapeño peppers, chopped
- 6 garlic cloves, peeled
- ¼ cup apple cider vinegar (this is not strictly Paleo, but many modern Paleo followers accept it as "legal" as it has many health benefits)
- 2 tablespoons organic honey
- 2 tablespoons Paleo-friendly fish sauce
- 1 teaspoon Himalaya salt
- 4 tablespoons tomato sauce (home-made)

Method: blend, cool down in a fridge and enjoy. This recipe makes about 1 cup of sriracha sauce.

Method of preparation:

1.Chop all the vegetables and shrimps as is mentioned in the ingredients list. Toss the vegetables in a salad bowl.

2.Now combine the palm sugar, almond butter, lime juice, sriracha sauce, coconut milk and fish sauce in a food processor. Process until the palm sugar breaks and you get a smooth salad dressing.

3.Add the cooked shrimps to the vegetables mixture after slitting those halfway lengthwise through the middle.

4.Add the palm sugar salad dressing to the shrimps and vegetables salad and mix well. Garnish with raw cashews, lime wedges and chopped scallions before serving.

Paleo Seafood Salad

Servings: 3-4
Preparation time: 12 hours

Ingredients:

- oz. (226.796 grams) of cooked baby shrimps, shelled and chopped
- 2/3 cup of homemade paleo mayonnaise
- oz. (226.796 grams) of sweet crab meat
- 2/3 cup of chopped celery
- 1/2 teaspoon of organic celery salt
- 1 cup of finely chopped white onion
- 1/2 teaspoon of garlic powder
- 1 tablespoon of hot sauce (you can use the one from the previous recipe)
- 2 tablespoons Dijon mustard
- 1/4 teaspoon of onion powder

Method of preparation:

1.Chop the celery and the white onion as required. Add the chopped shrimps and crab meat.

2.Add the rest of the ingredients and toss together to coat.

3.Transfer the salad to an air right refrigerator compatible container and serve the salad chilled within a few hours (or the next day). Perfect for those who like to have their food prepared in advance!

Bacon Brussels Salad

Servings: 10
Preparation time: 40 minutes

Ingredients:

- 6 whole slices of organic cooked bacon, chopped or crumbled
- 1 cup of grated paleo home-made cashew parmesan cheese*
- 1 whole orange
- 1 cup of almonds
- 1/2 cup olive oil
- 1 whole lemon
- 4 dozens of Brussels sprouts
- 1 large sized shallot, finely chopped
- A dash of black pepper
- Sea salt, to taste

*Vegan Paleo Parmesan Cheese is super easy to make. All you need is to blend: 1 cup of raw cashews with ¼ cup of nutritional yeast and a bit of Himalaya salt. No excuses now. Cutting out dairy is easy if you prepare yourself with the right ingredients.

Method of preparation:

1.Place the shallots in a bowl. Add the lemon and orange juice as well as olive oil while whisking the mixture constantly to prepare an emulsion. Transfer the emulsion to refrigerator and let sit for a few hours.
2.Cook the bacon slices in a skillet until crispy and all done. Crumble or cut the bacon slices into small bite sized pieces. Drain and set aside. Shave the Brussels sprouts and add the crumbled Paleo cheese and bacon pieces to the sprouts.
3.Process the almonds in a food processor.
4.Add the crumbled almonds and olive oil emulsion to the sprouts salad and toss well to combine. Enjoy!

Crabmeat Spinach Salad

Servings: 4
Preparation time: 10 minutes

Ingredients:

- 1/2 lb. (680.389 grams) of cooked crabmeat
- 2 bunch of spinach leaves, rinsed
- 2 large sized tomatoes, thinly sliced
- 2 pieces of hardboiled eggs, thinly sliced
- 1 Maui sweet onion, sliced thinly

Ingredients for salad dressing:

- 1 cup of fresh tomato puree
- 1 teaspoon of cayenne pepper
- 3 tablespoons of dry mustard powder (organic)
- 2 cup of flaxseed oil
- 1 tablespoon of ground black pepper
- 1 cup of freshly extracted lemon juice
- 1 large clove of garlic, peeled and minced
- 1 cup of paleo burgundy wine
- 1 tablespoon of black pepper

Method of preparation:

1.Blend the salad dressing ingredients and set aside.

2.Mix the crabmeat with spinach leaves pieces, sliced sweet onion, egg slices and tomato slices.

3.Add the required amount of salad dressing to the salad and toss lightly to coat and serve immediately. Enjoy!

Seared Scallops Salad with Arugula

Servings: 4
Preparation time: 15 minutes
Cooking time: 50-55 minutes

Ingredients:

- 1 lb. (453.592 grams) of sea scallops
- 2 garlic cloves, peeled and minced (you can also use garlic powder)
- 3oz. of baby arugula, rinsed and chopped
- 1 teaspoon of fresh lemon zest
- 4 tablespoons of olive oil
- 2 tablespoons of fresh lemon juice
- 1/4 teaspoon of ground black pepper
- 2 teaspoons of kosher salt

Method of preparation:

1.To prepare the salad dressing, combine the minced garlic with salt, black pepper and lemon zest with lemon juice. Whisk to combine well.

2.Now slowly and steadily add the olive oil while whisking continuously to form the dressing. Set aside the dressing to let the flavors marry for 15 minutes.

3.Toss the salad dressing with arugula. Set aside.

4.Rinse and dry the scallops. Season those with salt and pepper.

5.Heat up oil in a large skillet and place the seasoned scallops in it once the oil turns hot. Sear the scallops for 3-4 minutes or until golden browned. Flip the scallops and sear the other side for 1-2 minutes. Drain and set the scallops aside.

6.Serve the seared scallops over the arugula salad. Enjoy!

Yummy Sesame Beef Salad

Servings: 4
Preparation time: 20-25 minutes
Cooking time: 15-20 minutes

Ingredients:
- 2lbs. (907 grams) of ground beef or bison
- 2 tablespoons of paleo Worcestershire sauce
- 1 bunch of scallions, sliced
- 2 garlic cloves, peeled and minced
- 1 carrot, peeled and grated
- 1/2 head of red cabbage, sliced thinly into ribbons
- 2 tablespoons of coconut aminos
- 1/2 cup of fresh cilantro leaves, chopped
- oz. (226.8 grams) of fresh mixed greens of your choice
- A dash of cayenne pepper
- 1 tablespoons of sesame oil
- 2 tablespoons of sesame seeds
- Kosher salt, to taste
- 1 whole lime, juiced
- Some ground black pepper, to taste

Method of preparation:

1.Toast the sesame seeds until golden. Remove from hot pan and set aside to prevent the seeds from scorching.
2.Dump the ground beef in the same pan and cook until beef is browned and no longer in lumps. Add the garlic and cayenne pepper to the beef and stir to combine nicely.
3.Finally add the coconut aminos, salt, black pepper, lime juice and Worcestershire sauce to the beef. Give a nice stir to mix everything up thoroughly. Once done, turn off the heat and remove from pan.
4.Chop and slice the cabbage, carrot, and scallions. Add cilantro leaves. Toss the vegetables and mixed greens with sesame oil.

Top the vegetables and mixed greens with the browned beef and serve.

Sirloin Salad with Balsamic Vinaigrette

Servings: 2-4

Preparation time: 15 minutes

Cooking time: 5 minutes

Ingredients:
- 1/2 cup of bacon bits, fried
- 1/2 lb. (226.8 grams) of grass-fed sirloin, cooked and sliced
- 1/2 cup of fresh cherry tomatoes, halved
- 1/2 cup of almonds
- 1/2 cup of red onion rings
- 1/2 cup of dried cranberries
- Dressing:
- 4 tablespoons of coconut vinegar
- 3/4 cup of olive oil (extra virgin)
- 2 garlic cloves, peeled
- Salt, to taste
- Black pepper, to taste

Method of preparation:

1.Arrange all the salad ingredients side by side in a salad platter and place the cooked sirloin at the middle.

2.To prepare the dressing, process everything together (except for the oil) until a smooth dressing is formed. Add the extra virgin olive oil at the end while still processing the mixture.

3.Once everything is ready, serve the dressing beside the salad.

Avocado BLT Egg Salad

Servings: 3-4

Preparation time: 10 minutes

Cooking time: 10 minutes

Ingredients:

- 4 strips of bacon, cooked until crispy

- 1 whole avocado

- 1/2 cup of fresh scallions, chopped

- 6 hard-boiled eggs

- 2 teaspoon of ground garlic

- 1/2 teaspoon of Himalayan sea salt, more to taste

- 3/4th cup of grape tomatoes cut in halves

Method of preparation:

1.Combine the hard boiled eggs with avocado, sea salt and ground garlic. Do not mash the eggs completely.

2.Finally add the rest of the ingredients to the eggs mixture and serve immediately.

Bacon Fennel Salad with Grilled Peaches

Servings: 4-6
Preparation time: 30-40 minutes
Cooking time: 20-25 minutes

Ingredients:

- 1 cup of chopped fennel bulb
- 4 slices of bacon, cooked and chopped into small bits
- 1 tablespoon of melted coconut oil
- 3-4 ripe peaches
- 1 tablespoon of coconut oil
- 1/2 lb. (226.8 grams) of mixed salad greens
- A pinch of celtic sea salt

For the dressing:

- 4 whole dried dates, pitted
- 5 tablespoons of olive oil
- 1 strip of cooked bacon
- 2 tablespoons of bacon fat
- 2 tablespoons of coconut vinegar
- 1/4 teaspoon of celtic sea salt

Method of preparation:

1. Heat up 1 tablespoon of coconut oil in a skillet and drop the chopped fennel in it. Sauté the fennel until cooked and aromatic, for about 4-5 minutes. Once done, drain the fennel and set aside.
2. To prepare the grilled peaches, cut those in half and pit the halves.
3. Grease the cut side of the peach slices with remaining coconut oil and place on the grill. Grill the peaches lid-on over medium heat for 12-15 minutes or until the peaches turn tender and start falling apart.
4. To prepare the salad dressing, blend all the ingredients required until everything is processed and the dressing is smooth and lump free.

5.Toss the salad greens along with the salad dressing. Add the cooked bacon, grilled peach halves and fennel to the salad. Serve right away.

Back Ribs Cherry Cabbage Slaw

Servings: 4-6
Preparation time: 20-25 minutes
Cooking time:1 hour 30 minutes

Ingredients:

- 1 entire rack of pork ribs, cut in half crosswise

Spice rub:

- 1 tablespoon of ground ancho chiles
- 1 teaspoon of celery seed
- 1 tablespoon of dried thyme
- 1 teaspoon of ground mustard
- 1 tablespoon of garlic powder
- 1 teaspoon of cayenne
- 1 tablespoon of onion powder
- 1 teaspoon dried rosemary
- 1 tablespoon of smoked paprika
- 1 teaspoon of sea salt

Cherry cabbage slaw:

- 2 medium sized carrots, shredded
- 1/2 of a cabbage head, cored and thinly sliced
- Juice of 2 limes
- Zest of 2 limes
- 2 cups of fresh cherries, pitted and halved
- 1/2 of a red onion, peeled and thinly sliced
- 4 tablespoons of olive oil
- Sea salt
- Black pepper

Method of preparation:

1.Prepare spice rub by mixing all the ground spices together. Rub the salad rub over the pork ribs and transfer the ribs to a baking dish (add ¼ cup water).

2.Bake the pork ribs in a 325 degrees Fahrenheit (or: 160 Celsius) oven for 80-85 minutes. Once done, remove the pork from oven and set aside.

3.Set the grill to medium high and grill the ribs for 10-12 minutes or until the ribs are crispy.

4.Finally, toss the cabbage, cherries, onion and carrots with olive oil, lime zest, lime juice, sea salt and black pepper to prepare the slaw.

5.Serve the grilled ribs alongside the slaw.

Section 5

Paleo Fruit Salads

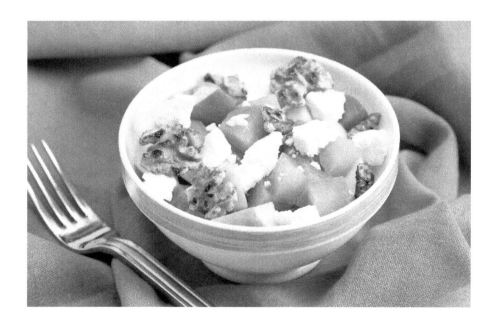

Pink Grapefruit with Avocado Salad

Servings: 4

Preparation time: 10 minutes

Ingredients:

- 2 whole avocados

- 1 tablespoon of extra virgin olive oil

- A pinch of sea salt

- 2 grapefruits

- 1 tablespoon of coconut vinegar

Method of preparation:

1.Slice the avocados in halves. Remove the pits and cut the avocado flesh into small cubes or slices.

2.Segment the grapefruits and add the pieces to the avocado chunks.

3.Whisk the coconut vinegar with some olive oil. Add sea salt and mix well. Pour over the salad and serve. Enjoy! This salad is extremely alkaline and will help you balance your pH.

Waldorf-ish Salad

Servings: 4-5
Preparation time: 10 minutes
Cooking time: 5 minutes

Ingredients:

- 3 medium sized organic red apples, cored and diced
- 1 1/2 teaspoon of organic maple syrup
- 3 stalks of celery, sliced on the bias
- 4 tablespoons of pecans
- 1 teaspoon of coconut butter
- 1 tablespoon of paleo apple cider vinegar
- 2 tablespoons of coconut cream
- A pinch of cayenne pepper
- Sea salt
- Ground black pepper, to taste

Method of preparation:

1.Melt the coco butter and add 1 teaspoon of maple syrup to it (use a small frying-pan). Drop the pecans in the mixture and stir energetically.

2.Cook for 3-4 minutes or until the pecans turn golden brown. Once done, drain and allow to cool down.

3.Slice and dice the celery and the apples. Place in a salad bowl.

4.Combine the remaining maple syrup with coconut cream, apple cider vinegar, cayenne pepper, salt and ground black pepper.

5.Drizzle salad dressing on top of salad, add the pecans and toss with salad. Enjoy!

<u>Simple Pear and Walnut Salad</u>

Servings: 4

Preparation time: 8-10 minutes

Ingredients:

- 1/2 cup of dried cherries

- 3/4th cup of walnuts, organic

- 2 ripe pears

- 5 cups of salad greens

- 2 tablespoons of coconut milk

- Juice of 2 lemons

Method of preparation:

1.Cut the pears into bite sized pieces and transfer to a salad bowl.

2.Add the walnuts, salad greens and dried cherries to the pears and toss nicely.

3.Serve the salad with coconut milk and lemon sauce or any other salad dressings of choice. Enjoy!

<u>Winter Fruit Salad</u>

Servings: 4

Preparation time: 10-15 minutes

Ingredients:

- 100 grams (3.5 oz.) of fresh rocket leaves
- 1/2 fresh lemon
- 2 blood oranges, peeled and halved horizontally
- 1.05 oz. (30 grams) of paleo cashew cheese (mentioned in previous recipes)
- 1 whole pomegranate, seeded
- A few small sprigs of mint, leaves separated
- Some olive oil

Method of preparation:

1.Rinse the rocket leaves. Drain and set aside. Peel and slice the oranges and then seed the pomegranate.

2.To prepare the dressing, whisk together lemon juice, salt and olive oil.

3.Toss the orange pieces and rocket leaves with the dressing and then transfer to serving plates.

4.Drop the pomegranate seeds and sprinkle over some paleo cheese on top and serve. Enjoy!

Papaya Avocado Slaw

Servings: 3-4

Preparation time: 10-15 minutes

Ingredients:

- 10 oz. (283.495 grams) of organic broccoli slaw

- 2 tablespoons of lemon juice

- 1 cup of ripe papaya, cubed

- 2 tablespoons of finely chopped fresh cilantro

- 1/2 avocado, peeled and chopped

- 1/2 tablespoon of paleo balsamic vinegar (not really Paleo, but accepted by many Paleo gurus due to its numerous health benefits)

Method of preparation:

1.Cut the papaya, avocado and chop the cilantro.

2.Mix all the ingredients together in a salad bowl. Serve and enjoy.

Grapes and Walnuts Salad

Servings: 8

Preparation time: 5 minutes

Ingredients:

- 2 lbs. (907 grams) of fresh grapes

- 1 cup raw walnut halves

- 2 tablespoons of olive oil

- 3 big avocados, peeled, pitted and diced

- 2 tablespoons of paleo red wine vinegar

Method of preparation:

1.Dump the grapes and the walnut in a large salad bowl. Add avocado pieces on top and toss the salad with some red wine vinegar and olive oil.

2.Refrigerate to chill and serve.

Strawberry with Prosciutto Salad

Servings: 2

Preparation time: 10 minutes

Cooking time: 5 minutes

Ingredients:

- 4 cups baby spinach
- 2 oz. (56.7 grams) of smoked almonds
- 2 cups sliced strawberries
- 2 oz. (56.7 grams) of crumbled paleo cheese (use the vegan cashew nut cheese recipe mentioned previously)
- 4 thin slices of prosciutto
- 4 tablespoons of paleo organic balsamic dressing

Method of preparation:

1.Broil the prosciutto slices on high for 5 minutes or until crispy. Cool down.

2.Slice the strawberries and transfer to a bowl. Add the spinach leaves to the strawberry slices.

3.Crumble the paleo cheese and prosciutto slices on top. Drizzle balsamic dressing on top and serve. Enjoy!

Pear Apple and Spinach Salad

Servings: 4
Preparation time: 10 minutes

Ingredients:

- 2 medium sized pears, peeled, cored and thinly sliced
- 6 cups of fresh baby spinach
- 1 cup of dried cranberries
- 2 medium sized apples, peeled, cored and sliced thinly
- 1/3 cup of olive oil
- 1 tablespoons of lemon juice
- Some Paleo mustard to taste
- A dash of ground black pepper
- 4 tablespoons of paleo apple cider vinegar
- 1 tablespoon of raw honey
- A dash of sea salt

Method of preparation:

1.Peel, core and slice the apples and pears as mentioned. Pour enough water over the fruit slices, so as to cover the fruits entirely up to the top with water. Place a small sized plate over the fruit slices, so as to make them remain submerged in the water.

2.Prepare the salad dressing by whisking apple cider vinegar with some olive oil, and honey. Add mustard, sea salt, lemon juice and pepper and whisk until there are no clumps in the mixture.

3.Combine the spinach and cranberries in a separate bowl. Drain the fruits and add those to the spinach and cranberries mixture.

4.Drizzle the salad dressing on top and serve. Enjoy!

Lemon Refreshing Fruit Salad

Servings: 4

Preparation time: 20 minutes

Ingredients:

- 2 large sized Fuji or Gala apples, peeled, cored and cubed

- 2 large sized navel oranges, peeled and sliced

- 2 large sized mangoes, peeled and cubed

- 2 teaspoons of finely grated fresh ginger

- 2 large sized red Bartlett pears

- 2 tablespoons of organic honey

- 1 pineapple, peeled, cored and cubed

- 4 tablespoons of fresh lemon juice

Method of preparation:

1.Peel and cut the apples, mangoes, pears, oranges and pineapple into small bite sized pieces or cubes.

2.Mix the lemon juice, grated ginger and honey in a bowl to prepare the salad dressing.

3.Pour the salad dressing over the salad and toss to finish the preparation.

197

Peach Nectarine and Strawberry Salad with Honey Lime Basil Syrup

Servings: 6

Preparation time: 10 minutes

Ingredients:

- 6 large sized strawberries
- 1 whole lime
- 1 tablespoon lime zest
- 3 white peaches
- 1 tablespoon of honey
- 3 large nectarines
- 1 tablespoon chopped fresh basil

Method of preparation:

1.Quarter the strawberries and cut the nectarines and peaches into bite sized pieces.

2.Prepare the syrup by mixing honey with basil and lime juice.

3.Mix all the fruits in a salad bowl. Sprinkle over some lemon zest and syrup to the salad.

4.Toss to mix and serve right away. Enjoy!

Strawberry Caprese Salad

Servings: 1
Preparation time: 5 minutes

Ingredients:
- 10 whole strawberries
- Extra virgin olive oil
- 3.5oz (100 g) of paleo vegan mozzarella cheese***
- Crushed black pepper (to taste)
- 15 fresh organic basil leaves

Method of preparation:
1.Quarter the strawberries and add the paleo mozzarella cheese.
2.Add the basil leaves and season the salad with black pepper.
3.Drizzle desired amount of olive oil over the salad. Toss the salad and serve to enjoy.

***Here's what you need to make Paleo mozzarella cheese:
- 1/2 cup of thick coconut milk
- 1 cup coconut butter, half-melted
- Half cup of melted coconut oil
- Nutritional yeast (4 tablespoons)
- A pinch of Himalaya salt
- Juice of 2 lemons
- 1 teaspoon of garlic powder (yummy!)
- Half cup of melted coconut oil

Blend all the ingredients adding melted coconut oil last. Blend again until 100% smooth.
Pour into a freezer-safe container and freeze for about 1 hour.
Serve with salads, enjoy!

Nutty Fruity Salad

Servings: 2

Preparation time: 10-12 minutes

Ingredients:

- 1 whole apple, cubed
- 1 whole banana, peeled and sliced
- 1 whole orange, cut into segments
- 1/4 of a pineapple, cut into cubes
- A handful of sunflower seeds
- 6-7 fresh strawberries, halved
- A handful of almonds
- A handful of organic pumpkin seeds

Method of preparation:

1.Peel and slice the banana, cut the apples and pineapples into cubes and segment the orange.

2.Transfer the chopped fruits to a salad bowl.

3.Add the nuts and seeds to the fruits and toss lightly to mix up. Serve immediately.

Simple Fruit Salad

Servings: 10

Preparation time: 30-40 minutes

Ingredients:

- 1 whole ripe papaya

- 8-10 lychees, pitted

- 1/2 watermelon, seeded and cut into cubes

- 3 whole mangoes, pitted and cubed

- 5 fresh kiwis, sliced

- 6 apricots, sliced

- 3-4 ripe bananas, sliced

- 2 teaspoons of paleo vanilla extract

- 2 teaspoons cinnamon powder

Method of preparation:

1.Dump all the fruit slices in a large sized salad bowl.

2.Drizzle the vanilla extract and add a dash of cinnamon powder to the salad. Toss the salad slightly and serve fresh.

<u>Simple Avocado Alkaline Salad</u>

Servings: 4

Preparation time: 10-15 minutes

Ingredients:

- 2 ripe avocados, mashed or cubed
- ½ of a red onion, peeled and chopped
- 1 whole ripe mango, cubed
- 1 teaspoon of fresh lime juice
- 1 garlic clove, peeled and minced
- ½ red onion, chopped
- A cup of cherry tomatoes, halved
- 1 whole jalapeño, deseeded and minced
- Fresh greens
- 1 Thai red chili, deseeded and minced (optional)
- A dash of avocado oil
- Sea salt, to taste

Method of preparation:

Cut and chop the vegetables and fruits. Mix everything up in a salad bowl and serve right away. Enjoy!

BONUS: SECTION 6 PALEO SALAD SAUCES AND CONDIMENTS

Aside from a few condiments and non-dairy Paleo solutions that I have mentioned in this book, I would love to introduce you to my favorite Paleo salad dressings and condiments. Spice up your salads and enjoy variety! Enjoy the creative Paleo ride and design a healthy lifestyle for you and your family.

Paleo Tahini Salad Dressing

Servings: 1/4th cup

Preparation time: 5 minutes

Ingredients:

- 2-3 tablespoons of Tahini (sesame seed butter)

- Some organic apple cider vinegar, to taste

- 1 whole lemon, juiced

- Ground black pepper, to taste

- 2 cloves of garlic

- Sea salt, to taste

Method of preparation:

1.Blend all the ingredients until well combined and smooth.

2.Add more water or apple cider vinegar to loosen out dressing, if required.

Orange Poppy Dressing

Servings: 2-3

Preparation time: 5-7 minutes

Ingredients:

- 1 tablespoons of paleo Dijon mustard

- 1 orange, juiced

- 1 tablespoon of poppy seeds

- Zest of 1 orange

- 1 whole garlic clove, smashed

- 1 teaspoon of paleo white wine vinegar

- 4 tablespoons of paleo mayonnaise

- 1/4th teaspoon of ground white pepper

- 1/4th teaspoon of Himalayan salt

Method of preparation:

1.Blend all the ingredients until you achieve smooth salad dressing.

2.Toss and serve with a yummy Paleo salad of your choice!

Chive and Hemp Oil Salad Dressing

Servings: 1 cup

Preparation time: 5 minutes

Ingredients:

- 1 tablespoon of hemp oil
- 1/2 teaspoon of raw honey
- 1 teaspoon of paleo red wine vinegar
- 1 tablespoon of finely chopped chives
- 1 clove fresh garlic, minced
- 1 tablespoon of extra virgin olive oil

Method of preparation:

1.Combine the red wine vinegar, extra virgin olive oil, hemp oil, chopped chives, honey and minced garlic in a bowl.

2.Whisk the mixture until everything is well combined and you get a smooth salad dressing. Serve with a yummy Paleo salad of your choice!

Maple Mustard Dressing

Servings: 4

Preparation time: 4-5 minutes

Ingredients:

- 2 teaspoons of organic maple syrup

- 1 tablespoon light olive oil

- Some black pepper to taste

- 2 tablespoons of organic Dijon mustard

Method of preparation:

1.Take the maple syrup in a small bowl and add Dijon mustard, olive oil and ground black pepper to the maple syrup.

2.Whisk the mixture in the bowl to prepare the salad dressing.

3.Serve with a yummy Paleo salad of your choice!

Carrot Ginger Salad Dressing

Servings: 6

Preparation time: 6-8 minutes

Ingredients:

- ½ lb. (226.8 grams) of peeled and chopped carrots,
- 4 tablespoons of paleo apple cider vinegar
- 1 tablespoon of coconut aminos
- ¼ cup of fresh ginger, peeled and chopped
- ½ cup olive oil
- 1 chopped onion (small)
- 1/8 teaspoon of sea salt
- 1 tablespoon of sesame oil

Method of preparation:

1.Peel and coarsely chop the carrots. Dump the carrots in food processor and process until the carrots are nicely processed and turn into a paste.

2.Add the coconut aminos, sesame oil, chopped onions, ginger, vinegar and sea salt to the carrots. Process again until the dressing is loosened a bit. Then add some olive oil to it. Process well to combine and serve with a yummy Paleo salad of your choice!

Creamy Citrus Almond Dressing

Servings: 1

Preparation time: 5 minutes

Ingredients:

- 1 tablespoon of fresh orange juice

- 1 teaspoon of organic almond butter

- Salt, to taste

- 1 tablespoon of avocado oil

- Black pepper, to taste

- 1/4 teaspoon of minced garlic

Method of preparation:

1.Peel and mince the garlic cloves.

2.Blend in a blender. Serve with a yummy Paleo salad of your choice.

Tomato Cilantro Dressing

Servings: 4

Preparation time: 5-7 minutes

Ingredients:

- 1 tomato

- 1/4 cup of olive oil

- 2 cloves of garlic, peeled

- 1/2 small red onion

- A handful of fresh cilantro

- 2 green onions

- Sea salt, to taste

- Black pepper, to taste

Method of preparation:

1.Rinse all the vegetables and set aside.

2.Blend all the veggies until everything is fairly nicely processed.

3.Do not make the dressing too smooth. Serve with a yummy Paleo salad of your choice!

__Catalina Dressing__

Servings: 1 cup

Preparation time: 5 minutes

Ingredients:

- 2 tablespoons of fresh tomato paste
- ½ cup of olive oil
- 1 teaspoon of Paleo mustard
- 4 tablespoons of raw apple cider vinegar
- Half teaspoon of paprika
- 1 tablespoon of raw honey
- 1teaspoon of onion granules
- 1/2 teaspoon garlic granules
- 1/4 teaspoon of chili powder
- A pinch of black pepper

Method of preparation:

1.Combine all the ingredients and whisk well.

2.Once done, store the salad dressing in a container or jar and serve with any salad of choice.

BONUS Alkaline Paleo Salad Recipes for Optimal Health & Nutrition

Shredded Chicken with Stir Fried Alkaline Vegetables

Servings: 2-3
Preparation time: 20 minutes
There's nothing more delicious and nutritious than chicken. Combine it with alkaline vegetables and you get the most energy filled lunch.

Ingredients:
- 1 tablespoon olive oil
- 1 bowl of chopped Zucchini
- 1 bowl shredded cabbage
- 1 bowl of yellow, red and green bell peppers
- Two onions roughly sliced
- 3-4 Garlic cloves
- 1 bowl of carrots
- 1 tablespoon almonds
- 1 cup (250gr) shredded chicken (you can use some leftovers)
- Salt to taste

Preparation

1.Chop zucchini, bell peppers, carrots and set them aside. Cut thin slices of garlic cloves.
2.Take a sauce pan and put one tablespoon of olive oil in it. Put it on slow heat and then add sliced garlic to it. 3.
3.When the garlic turns light brown, add onions and sauté for a while.
4.Later add all the sliced vegetables and fry them for about 5 minutes on medium heat.
5.Now add the chicken sprinkle some salt as per your taste and cover it with a lid.
6.Stir-fry for about 10 minutes, the cool down and serve.

Serving: Serve in a colored plate and decorate it with a slice of pineapple on the side. To add some more crunch to it, you can use chopped parsley or spinach, deep fry it and sprinkle it on top of this dish. Alternatively you can always add some fresh greens.

Easy Salad Wrap

Servings: 2-3

Preparation time: 15 minutes

Chicken, as we all know contains substantial amount of proteins. Be sure to use organic, free range chicken for maximum benefits.

Ingredients

- 4-5 iceberg or Romanian lettuce leaves
- 2-3 avocados
- 2 ripe tomatoes
- 1 chopped onion + 1 for garnishing
- 1 cup shredded chicken
- Some parsley
- Some salt to taste
- 1 pinch of pepper powder
- 1 teaspoon lime juice
- 2 sheets of gluten-free paleo-friendly tortillas

Preparation

1.The first step is to mash the ripe avocadoes properly. Slice the tomatoes, onion, parsley and Romanian lettuce.

2.Now put these ingredients in a large bowl and add pieces of chicken to it. Squeeze some lime juice into it. Add salt, some pepper powder and toss it well.

3.Take tortilla sheets and place them on a tray. Now carefully fill them with the salad mixture and roll them. You can secure the roll with a toothpick.

Serving

Take a couple of lettuce leaves and place them on a large white dish, one on top of the other. Now place the tortillas on top of them and serve. You can insert a couple of olives or cherry tomatoes on the tip of the toothpick to make it look more appealing. You can serve this wrap with a coconut yogurt and mint dip.

Paleo Salmon Salad

Salmon is an excellent, lean source of protein as well as healthy omega acids.

It is low in sodium which makes it a nice addition to the alkaline diet. My Paleo style husband loves it too. This salad is really quick to prepare, raw and high in nutrients. A recommend for Alkaline Paleo fans as well.

Servings: 4
Preparation time: max 20 minutes

Ingredients:
- A few strips of smoked salmon, cut into smaller pieces
- Half cup of almonds
- 2 carrots, peeled (unless organic) and sliced
- 1 cucumber, peeled and sliced
- 1 onion, minced
- 2 cups of baby spinach
- 4 big tomatoes, sliced
- 2 garlic cloves, minced
- 2 big peppers, chopped
- Optional: ¼ of iceberg lettuce
- Juice of 1 lemon and olive oil
- Himalaya salt and rosemary herb

Preparation:
1. Wash all the ingredients, peel and chop.
2. Mix in a big bowl.
3. Sprinkle over some olive oil and lemon juice.
4. Add Himalaya salt to taste.
5. Enjoy, we do!

Mediterranean Omega Salad with Tuna

Another quick recipe inspired by traditional Southern European Diet.

Servings: 4

Preparation time: max 10 minutes

Ingredients:

- Half iceberg lettuce, washed, dried and chopped
- 1 cup of baby spinach, washed, dried and chopped
- 1 big avocado, washed, peeled, pitted and chopped
- 2 cans of tuna
- 2 tomatoes, washed and sliced
- 2 carrots, washed, peeled (unless organic) and sliced
- 2 cucumbers, washed, peeled and sliced
- 1 big onion, minced
- 2 garlic cloves, peeled and minced
- Olive oil
- Juice of 2 lemons
- Optional: 2 tablespoons of soy lecithin granules (equals to better memory and concentration- great for both kids and adults)

Instructions:

1.Simply mix all the veggies and pasta in a big bowl.

2.Sprinkle over some olive oil and lemon juice.

3.Add salt to taste. Enjoy!

Easy Veggie Salad

Servings: 2

Preparation time: max 15 minutes

Ingredients:

- 2 big apples, peeled, pitted and chopped
- 1 avocado, peeled, pitted and chopped
- 2 tomatoes, slices
- 2 carrots, peeled and sliced
- 1 big pepper (green, red or orange), sliced
- Juice of 1 lemon
- Olive oil
- Himalaya Salt
- 1 cup of green olives, pitted
- A few raisins

Instructions:

1.Mix all the ingredients in a bowl.

2.Add olive oil, lemon juice and Himalaya salt.

3.Don't forget about olives and raisins! An excellent combination.

__Color Stir Fry__

Servings: 4

Preparation time: max 20 minutes

Ingredients:

- A few slices of salmon, bacon or other protein of your choice
- 1 big onion, peeled and minced
- 2 garlic cloves, peeled and minced
- Coconut oil
- A few tablespoons of coconut milk
- A few big peppers (green, red and yellow), I usually go for 6 big peppers of mixed colors
- 2 zucchini
- Himalayan Salt

Preparation:

1.In a saucepan, heat up a few tablespoons of coconut oil.

2.Add garlic and onions and stir for a few minutes.

3.Add salmon (or bacon). Fry for a few minutes.

4.Add salt and a bit of coconut milk. Lower the heat.

5.Add chopped veggies and stir-fry until soft (low heat, 15 minutes).

6.Serve with a few lime or lemon slices.

7.Enjoy!

Carrots Aperitif

This is a fantastic alkaline aperitif...

Servings: 2

Preparation time: max 10 minutes

Ingredients:

- 3, 4 carrots, (cut in smaller sticks)

- 1 cucumber

- 1 avocado

- 2 tomatoes

- 2 tablespoons of coconut oil

- Himalayan salt

Preparation:

1.Blend avocado + tomatoes + cucumber.

2.Add some coconut oil and mix.

3.Add salt and pepper to taste.

4.Serve with carrot sticks. Cucumber sticks or radishes are also great.

5.Enjoy, we love this quick recipe when awaiting our main dish!

6.OPTIONAL- you can use it as raw alkaline salad dressing for other salads of your choice

Book 3 Alkaline Diet

Soup Recipes-

Supercharge Your Health, Beat Inflammation, and Lose Weight!

100% Plant-Based

By Elena Garcia

Introduction

Welcome to the *world of alkaline soup recipes,* where it's all about healthy and nutritious alkaline diet recipes that are easy to prepare and will give you the energy you deserve. They are perfect for all occasions, offer a variety of taste, are jam-packed with minerals and vitamins to rejuvenate all the cells of your beautiful body, help you have more energy for life, beat inflammation, and if desired, lose weight.

Most people already know that eating more veggies and natural, plant-based foods are good for them. But the question, "OK, so what am I going to eat to feel satisfied?" more often than not turns into procrastination and the big problem of not knowing how to turn theory into practice.

This is why I created this book- to make it simple, doable, and fun for you! Some soup recipes I created are raw food recipes and can also be consumed as smoothies, and there are also slow cooker recipes and much more.

All of them are comforting, healing, energizing, and perfect all year long. While this book and its recipes focus more on the plant-based approach, this book is not only for vegans and vegetarians. Everyone can benefit from it!

This book is for you if:

- You feel like you want to have more energy without depending on caffeine or energy drinks.
- You want to add some easy and healthy recipes to your collection.- You are vegan/vegetarian and want to add an alkaline twist to your nutrition.

- You want to lose weight without feeling deprived and without thinking too much about calories.
- You would like to reduce animal products from your diet but are not too sure what to eat (or how to make your food taste great).
- You want to transition towards a natural, wholesome, plant-based, anti-inflammatory diet.
- You don't want to spend hours in the kitchen, and as with most people in this busy day and age, you want to be able to save your time, yet still have delicious, healthy, home-cooked meals whenever you want.

The Alkaline Diet- The Common Sense Approach

Ok, so you got this book entitled "Alkaline Soups," and you already know it's something healthy. But perhaps you don't really know what "alkaline" means, or maybe you find it confusing (there is so much conflicting info out there).
The alkaline diet is a lifestyle that encourages you to give your body the nourishment it needs so that it can work for you at its optimal level without feeling too exhausted or acidic. Too much acidity in the body leads to depression, sickness, and obesity.

Dr. Robert O' Young, Director of Research at the pH Miracle Living Center, says that your fat may be protecting your very life against the acidity in your body. He goes on to make this bold statement:

"There is only one disease: the constant acidification of the body."

What this means is that every disease, including excess weight, is because of a body that is too acidic. These things can make your body too acidic: processed foods, sugar, gluten and yeast, too much meat and animal products, stress, alcohol, tobacco, drugs, caffeine, and pollution.
If you attend to the root cause of the problem by implementing a lifestyle rich in alkaline-forming foods that are full of nutrients, it will naturally take care of what plagues you.

*****
Before we dive into complicated pH discussions, here is one thing to understand:
- The alkaline diet is not about changing or "raising" your pH. This is where many alkaline guides go wrong. You see, our body is smart

enough to self-regulate our pH for us no matter what we eat. Unfortunately, when you constantly bombard your body with acid-forming foods (for example processed foods, fast food, alcohol, sugar, and even too much meat), you torture your body with incredible stress. Because it has to work harder to maintain that optimal pH.

Here's simple example...

Imagine you immerse yourself in a bath filled with ice. You say, hey, my body can self-regulate its optimal temperature, right? And yes, it can. But it will eventually collapse and you will get ill. The same happens with nutrition and our blood pH. You can spend years indulging in toxic, processed, acid-forming foods that only deprive your body of its vital nutrients, saying: "My body will self-regulate its optimal blood pH".
And again, it will, but sooner or later it will give up and manifest a disease. It will accumulate fat as its natural defense function to protect your body from over-acidity. We don't want to end up there, right?

So, to sum up, the alkaline diet is a natural, holistic system, a nutritional lifestyle that advocates consumption of fresh, unprocessed foods that are rich in nutrients. These are called alkaline foods, and they help your body stimulate its optimal healing functions. Yes! A healthy body needs nutrients, and fresh fruits and vegetables are great for that.

The problem is that nowadays, most diets are filled with acid-forming foods that eventually make it hard for the body to regulate its optimal, healthy blood pH, and artificial sweeteners do the same. Acidosis is very common in this day and age thanks to things we drink as well: coffee, alcohol, and sodas all have an acidic effect on our bodies. Not to mention the chemicals many people take in through things like smoking and drugs (even prescription drugs have this effect).

There are many ways that you could become acidic. Eating acid forming foods, stress, taking in too many toxins, and bodily processes all cause acidity in the body. Our internal systems try to balance themselves out and bring pH up with the help of the alkaline minerals that we ingest through our diet. If we do not take in a higher percentage of alkaline than acidic foods, we can become too acidic.

When you are acidic, it makes every process that your body normally does much more difficult or impossible for it to accomplish. We cannot properly absorb the beneficial nutrients we need from our food. Our cells are not able to produce energy efficiently. Our bodies are not able to fix damaged cells correctly. We will not be able to detoxify. Fatigue and illness will drag you down. Sounds horrible, doesn't it? Here are some signs that you are overly acidic.

-Feeling tired all the time. You have no physical or mental drive at all.

-You always feel cold or get sick easily.

-You are depressed or just feel "blah" all the time for no real reason.

-You get headaches for no apparent reason.

-You get watery eyes or inflamed eyelids.

-Your teeth are sensitive and may crack or chip.

-Your gums are inflamed and you are susceptible to canker sores.

-You have recurring bouts with throat problems including tonsillitis.

-Acidic stomach with acid indigestion and reflux is always an issue.

-Your fingernails crack, split, and break.

-You have super dry hair that sheds and is hay-like with split ends.

-You have dry, ashy skin.

-Your skin breaks out in acne or is irritated when you sweat.

-You get leg cramps and spasms.

Of course, remember that whenever you experience any health/medical conditions, you need to see your doctor first and get a checkup.
We do not offer any medical advice. This is just a simple recipe guide to get you inspired to create a healthy lifestyle.

Many people complain that this diet is hard to follow.
But the way we see it is this: it's perfect! Plus, it's not a diet, it's a lifestyle.
What we really like about it is that you don't have to be 100% perfect. It's enough to be 80% awesome and 20% relaxed. You can even swap the 80/20 rule for 70/30 rule, meaning that about 70% of your diet should be fresh, nutrient-dense alkaline-forming foods, and the remaining 30% can be acid- forming foods (however, they still should be fresh and organic, for example grass-fed meat or organic eggs, or some gluten-free grains and legumes).

Many alkaline diet and lifestyle lovers decide to go vegan and we often get asked by our readers:
In order to get alkaline, do I have to go vegan?
We believe it's totally up to you. Alkaline diet is pretty vegan in its design, and alkaline and vegan concepts very often overlap.
And yes, many people go alkaline and use it as a starting point to eventually go fully vegan. Again, it's up to you.

I just want to give you more than enough of information, inspiration, and motivation so that you create your own way, something that works for you.

The most important thing is to do what works for you. All you need to keep in mind is to aim to eat 70-80% alkaline and try to eat more vegan/plant-based, even if you are not fully vegan.
The recipe section will give you some ideas!
For the most part, as a general rule, green veggies, many fruits, lentils, and seeds/nuts are considered alkaline. Animals, their byproducts, gluten, and sugar-containing foods are generally acidic.

What are alkaline foods? Is it about their pH?
No, luckily, it's much easier. We don't care about the food's pH in its natural form. All we care about is the effect that the food has on the body after it has been consumed and metabolized. For example, lemons, grapefruits and limes are considered alkaline-forming foods.

What? Elena? Are you out of your mind? Everyone knows lemons are acidic...

Well, let me repeat. Lemons are acidic as far as their taste and pH in their natural state are concerned. But they are full of alkaline minerals and low in sugar, which makes them alkaline-forming foods.

At the same time, oranges contain more sugar, which makes them less alkaline-forming.

Let us repeat:
Some charts determine acidity or alkalinity of the food before it is consumed, and others (like the ones we follow and recommend) are more interested in the effect the food has on the body after it has been consumed.
It's really that simple!

As a general rule, alkaline foods are:
- Rich in minerals and vitamins
- Fresh, not packaged
- Not fermented
- Low in sugar (all kinds of sugar are acid-forming)
- Plant-based
- Mostly raw or slightly cooked
- Caffeine-free
- Chemical-free
- Provide hydration

As a general rule, acid-forming foods are:
- Full of chemicals
- Low in nutrients
- High in sugar
- Contain caffeine, alcohol, or toxins
- Processed
- Packaged
- Fermented
- Contain artificial ingredients
- Animal byproducts

So let's have a look at the food lists. We think that after our intro, it will be easier for you to understand the difference between alkaline and acid forming foods, even without looking at the charts.

One more thing- we base our food lists on Doctor Young's latest research.

We know it is quite confusing to see so many different charts online. We have been there.

The reason why so many other charts show such disparity is because they base their classifications on the readings for the so called PRAL, which stands for Potential Renal Acid Load research. Unfortunately, this is not a reliable source of practical information for us.

Why?

Well, PRAL tests burn the food at an extreme temperature and then take a read of the 'ash' that is left behind and what its pH is.

While this will give a read of its alkalinity from the mineral content of the food, by burning it at such a high temperature, they also burn away sugar. And sugar is very acid-forming.

That is why on some charts high sugar fruits are listed as super alkaline. Now, we are not saying that fruits are bad for you, most fruits are neutral or mildly acid forming and great as a natural snack or a part of a balanced diet. But they are not as alkalizing as most veggies are.

Some charts determine acidity or alkalinity on the food before it is consumed, while others, like the ones we list below, are more interested in the effect the food has on the body after it has been consumed.

ALKALIZING VEGETABLES
Asparagus
Broccoli
Chili
Pepper
Zucchini
Dandelion
Snow peas
Green beans
String beans
Runner beans
Spinach
Kale
Wakame
Kelp
Collards
Chives
Endive
Chard
Cabbage
Sweet Potato
Mint
Ginger
Coriander
Basil
Brussels sprouts
Cauliflower
Carrot
Beetroot
Eggplant

Garlic
Onion
Parsley
Celery
Cucumber
Watercress
Lettuce
Peas
Broad beans
New potato
Pumpkin
Radish

ALKALIZING FRUITS
Avocado
Tomato
Lemon
Lime
Grapefruit
Fresh coconut
Pomegranate

ALKALIZING PROTEIN
Almonds
Chestnuts
Millet
Protein powders (we love hemp)

ALKALINE OILS
Avocado oil
Coconut oil
Flax oil
Udo's oil
Olive oil

Other:
Alkaline water
GMO-free tofu (neutral)
Fresh goat and almond milk
Herbal tea
Buckwheat pasta

ALKALINE SUPERFOODS:
Wheatgrass
Barley grass
Kamut grass
Dog grass
Shave grass
Oat grass
Soy sprouts
Alfalfa sprouts
Amaranth sprouts
Broccoli sprouts
Fenugreek sprouts
Kamut sprouts
Mung Bean sprouts
Quinoa sprouts
Radish sprouts
Spelt sprouts

ALKALINE-FRIENDLY BREADS:
Sprouted bread
Sprouted wraps
Gluten/Yeast-free breads and wraps

ALKALIZING SWEETENERS
- Stevia (natural)

ALKALIZING SPICES & SEASONINGS
Chili peppers
Cinnamon
Curry
Ginger
Herbs
Sea salt

ALKALIZING NUTS AND SEEDS
Almonds
Coconut
Flax Seeds
Pumpkin seeds
Sesame seeds
Sunflower seeds

ACID SWEETENERS

Carob, corn syrup, sugar
ACID BEVERAGES
Alcohol, coffee, soda

ACID TOXINS AND DRUGS
All drugs, weed killers, insecticides, tobacco

ACID MEAT:
Bacon
Beef
Clams
Corned beef
Eggs
Lamb
Lobster
Mussels
Organ meats
Venison
Fish
Oyster
Pork
Rabbit
Sausage
Scallops
Shellfish
Shrimp
Tuna
Turkey
Veal
MIDLY ACID-FORMING/NEUTRAL FRUITS:
Apple
Apricot
Currants
Dates
Grapes
Mango
Peach
Pear
Prunes
Raisins
Raspberries
Strawberries
Tropical fruits

Cantaloupe
Cranberries
Honeydew melon
Orange
Pineapple
Plum

ACID-FORMING DAIRY AND EGGS
Butter
Cheese
Milk
Whey
Yogurt
Cottage cheese
Ice cream
Sour cream
Soy cheese
Eggs

MIDLY ACID-FORMING NUTS AND SEEDS
Cashews
Peanuts
Pecans
Pistachios
Walnuts
Brazil nuts
Chestnuts
Hazelnuts
Macadamia nuts

ACID-FORMING OILS
Cooked oil
Solid oil (margarine)
Oil exposed to heat
Light or air

ACID-FORMING DRINKS
Alcohol
Black tea
Coffee
Carbonated water
Pasteurized juice

Cocoa
Energy drinks
Sports drinks
Colas
Tap water
Milk
Green tea
Decaffeinated drinks
Flavored water

ACID-FORMING SAUCES
Mayonnaise
Ketchup
Mustard
Soy Sauce
Pickles
Vinegar
Tabasco
Tamari
Wasabi

Other ACID-FORMING FOODS:
Mushrooms
Miso
White breads and pastas
Rice and noodles
Chocolate
Chips
Pizza
Biscuits
Cigarettes
Drugs
Candy

There is debate on several items as to whether or not they are alkalizing or acidifying. Many charts lists them as neutral, and this is what we believe makes sense. The good thing about the alkaline lifestyle is that we do not have to eat 100 percent alkaline. As long as we are taking in MOSTLY alkalizing foods, we are still on track! Here are some of the debated foods:

- Apple cider vinegar

- Brazil nuts
- Brussels sprouts
- Buckwheat
- Cashews
- Chicken
- Corn
- Cottage Cheese
- Eggs
- Flax
- Green tea
- Honey
- Kombucha
- Lima beans
- Potatoes
- Pepitas
- Quinoa
- Sauerkraut
- Soy
- Squash
- Sunflower seeds
- Tomatoes

Use charts as a guide, but don't worry too much if you find it difficult to memorize or if you have doubts whether your favorite food is alkaline enough. I, Elena, keep one of my 'alkaline charts' in my wallet at all times to reference at the grocery store!

We also have easy printable charts that you can download at no cost.

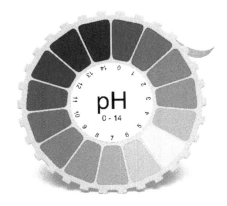

www.YourWellnessBooks.com/charts

Problems with your download?
Email us at: elenajamesbooks@gmail.com

The entire focus of the alkaline diet is to give your body the nourishment and healing tools it needs to MAINTAIN that optimal 7.365 pH almost effortlessly.

Slow Cooker Recipes

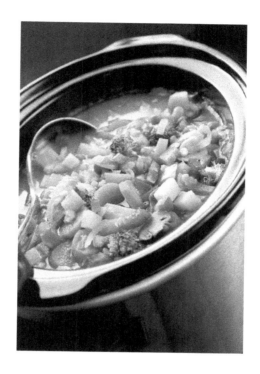

Butternut Squash Soup

This recipe is quick and easy. All you have to do is throw everything in the slow cooker and forget it. Your house will also end up smelling great. This is great for motivation and will inspire you to carry on your healthy lifestyle.

Servings: 6
Ingredients:

- Pepper
- Himalayan salt
- Optional: a few drops of stevia to sweeten
- ½ tsp /2 ½ ml cinnamon
- 2 14 oz. cans/784 g low-sodium vegetable broth
- 1 large chopped apple
- ¼ tsp /1 ¼ ml nutmeg
- 1 medium chopped butternut squash
- 3 medium chopped carrots
- 1 medium chopped onion

Chickpeas:

- 1/8 tsp /7/8 ml salt
- ¼ tsp /1 ¼ ml cinnamon
- 15 oz. can /420 g chickpeas
- 1 tbsp. /15 ml coconut oil

Instructions:
1.Add the fruits and vegetables to the slow cooker.

2.Top with the broth. Set for six hours on low.

3.After the veggies are soft, puree everything with an immersion blender. Stir in all the seasonings and add pepper and salt to your taste.

4.As the soup cooks, is the perfect time to fix the chickpeas.

5.The oven should be at 375.

6.Rinse the chickpeas and dry them.

7.Make sure to take off their skin.

8.Mix all the chickpea seasonings together and toss in the chickpeas.

9.Place them on a baking sheet and bake 40 to 45 minutes. Be sure to stir every 15 minutes. Serve the soup with the chickpeas. Enjoy

Quinoa White Chili

In the mood for a healthy, comforting, and cozy food? How about getting some detox along with some tasty comfort food? This recipe should fit the criteria very well. Do some quick prep work, throw everything in the slow cooker, and forget it. When you are ready to have a big bowl of this, squeeze some lime into your bowl and scatter a bit of cilantro over the top.

Servings: 6 - 8
Ingredients:

- Lime wedges
- Cilantro
- 2 15-oz. /420 g cans cannellini beans, drained
- 4 cups /960 ml low-sodium vegetable broth
- 1 tsp /5 ml salt
- 2 tsp /10 ml ground cumin
- 2 cloves garlic, minced
- ¼ tsp /1 ¼ ml paprika
- ¼ tsp /1 ¼ ml ground cloves
- ¾ cup /720 ml uncooked quinoa, rinsed with cold water, drained well
- 1 medium chopped onion
- 1 tsp /5 ml oregano
- 1 tbsp. /15 ml olive oil
- 2 medium poblano peppers
- 1 medium bell pepper, chopped
- Tabasco sauce to taste

Instructions:
1. Roast the poblano first. Oven needs to be on broil.
2. Move oven rack as close to broiler as possible.
3. Wash and dry the pepper and put on baking sheet.
4. Put in oven on broil for two to three minutes until black.
5. Flip them over.
6. Cook until blackened and blistered. Keep an eye on them: you want them blackened, not burnt.
7. Remove and place in brown paper bag to sweat.
8. Heat up a pan with oil.
9. Cook bell peppers and onions until soft.

10.Add spices.

11.Deglaze pan with broth.

12.Pour into slow cooker.

13.Add rest of broth, quinoa, beans, and Tabasco.

14.Peel skin off poblano and remove stem.

15.Chop and put into slow cooker. Mix together.

16.Allow to cook for about nine hours on low. Taste and enjoy!

Italian Bean Soup

This soup has the flavors of Italian sausage but without the meat.

This makes it a healthy and tasty meal for any day of the week. It's gluten-free, vegetarian, and vegan-friendly.

Why not experiment with plant-based foods?

Servings: 6
Ingredients:

- Pepper
- Salt
- 1 tbsp. /15 ml fennel seeds
- 2 tsp /10 ml oregano
- ¼ tsp /1 ¼ ml red pepper flakes
- 1 small chopped onion
- 2 celery ribs, chopped
- 3 medium chopped carrots
- 1 lb. /454 g dry Great Northern Beans
- 2 tsp /10 ml garlic powder

Instructions:

1.Add carrots, onions, celery, beans, spices except salt and pepper, and five cups cold water to cooker.

2.Set for five hours on high.

3.Add more water to give the soup the thickness you want. Add pepper and salt to taste. Serve and enjoy.

Black Bean Stew

This stew is so easy to throw together. Your house will end up smelling great, and there will also be leftovers to enjoy later in the week. Have fun with your toppings.

Servings: 6 - 8
Ingredients:

- Pepper
- Salt
- 1 - 2 dried chipotle peppers
- ¾ cup /720 ml uncooked quinoa, rinsed
- 1 cinnamon stick
- 3 minced garlic cloves
- 1 chopped green bell pepper
- cups /1.68 l water
- 1 medium chopped red onion
- 1 lb. /454 g dried black beans, rinsed, cleaned, and soaked overnight
- 2 tsp /10 ml chili powder
- 1 chopped red bell pepper
- ¼ cup /240ml fresh cilantro
- 1 28-oz. /784 g can diced tomatoes
- 1 tsp /5 ml coriander powder

Toppings:

- Avocado
- Lime wedges
- Thinly sliced green onions
- Cilantro

Instructions:
1.Add all ingredients except salt to the slow cooker.
2.Stir.
3.Set for nine hours on low.
4.After the beans are soft, add salt.
5.Remove chipotles and cinnamon stick.
6.Spoon into bowls and serve with toppings of your choice.

Red Pepper and Corn Chowder

This creamy chowder is healthy, comforting, and easy. It is much lighter than the usual version, but with smoky and sweet notes. It is packed full of flavor.

Servings: 4 - 6
Prep Time: 30 minutes
Ingredients:

- Pepper
- Salt
- 2 tbsp. /30 ml olive oil
- 4 cups /.95 L frozen sweet corn kernels, divided
- ½ tsp /2 ½ ml paprika
- 1 medium chopped red bell pepper
- 1 tsp /5 ml cumin
- 3 medium chopped Yukon Gold potatoes
- 1 medium chopped onion
- 1 cup /240 ml almond or coconut milk
- 1/8 tsp /7/8 ml cayenne pepper
- 4 cups /.95 L vegetable broth

Topping:

- Corn kernels
- Chopped scallions
- Chopped red bell pepper

Instructions:
1. Heat oil in a pan.
2. Add onion and cook until soft.
3. Place in slow cooker with bell pepper, a cup of corn, potatoes, spices, and broth.
4. Cook for nine hours on low.
5. After the potatoes are soft, puree everything with an immersion blender.
6. Stir in 3 cups of corn and almond or soy milk.
7. Cook an additional 30 minutes on low until warm.
8. Add pepper and salt to taste. Serve with toppings of your choice.

Farro Chili

This chili is quick and easy with spices that are easily adjusted to your unique tastes. It is filled with plenty of veggies, farro, and beans.

Servings: 6 - 8
Ingredients:

- Pepper
- 3 cups /720 ml low-sodium vegetable broth
- Himalayan Salt
- 1 ½ tbsp. /22.5 ml chili powder
- 1 15 oz. /420 g can pinto beans, rinsed and drained
- 2-14oz cans //784 g fire-roasted tomatoes, diced
- 1 chopped green pepper
- 1 pkg. sliced mushrooms
- 1 15 oz. /420 g can black beans, rinsed and drained
- 1 chopped orange pepper
- 2 tsp /10 ml garlic powder
- 1 medium chopped red onion
- 1 15 oz. /420 g can kidney beans, rinsed and drained
- 2 tsp /10 ml cumin
- 1 cup /240 ml farro, rinsed and drained
- 1 to 3 chipotle peppers in adobo sauce, chopped

Toppings:

- Sliced green onions
- Cilantro
- Avocado

Instructions:
1. Add all ingredients to the slow cooker. Stir.
2. Set for eight hours on low.
3. Veggies should be tender and liquid slightly thickened.
4. Season with pepper and salt.
5. Serve with toppings of your choice.

Vegetable Barley Soup

Barley absorbs liquids quickly, so adjust the liquid if you are planning on cooking this on high. This will also freeze well. Do not cook the chard at first. Add it at the end or if you are eating this later when reheating.

Servings: 6
Ingredients:

- Pepper
- Salt
- 1 small bunch Swiss chard
- sprigs fresh thyme
- ½ cup /120 ml barley (not the quick-cooking kind)
- 2 medium parsnips, chopped
- 1 small chopped rutabaga
- 2 celery stalks, chopped
- 1 large chopped onion
- 1 clove garlic, minced

Instructions:
1.Tie thyme with butcher's twine.
2.Add 8 cups water, barley, thyme, rutabaga, onion, garlic, celery, parsnips, pepper, and salt.
3.Cover. Set for 6 hours on low.
4.Make sure that the barley is tender.
5.When there is 10 minutes left on the timer, take out the thyme. Turn to high. Add Swiss chard, cover and cook until tender about 5 minutes.

Vegetable Stew

Carrots and turnips will turn sweet and soft as they cook slowly.

Servings: 6
Ingredients:

- Pepper
- Salt
- 1 zucchini, chopped
- 4 large carrots, sliced diagonally in 2-inch pieces
- ¼ tsp /1 ¼ ml red pepper flakes
- 1 15 oz. can /420 g chickpeas, drained
- 2 medium turnips, peeled and chopped into 1-inch cubes
- ½ tsp /2 ½ ml cumin
- 1 large diced onion
- 1 cup /240 ml vegetable broth
- 2 cloves minced garlic
- 1 14 oz. can /392 g diced tomatoes

Instructions:

1.Add tomatoes and liquid, garlic, onion, turnips, carrots, broth, pepper flakes, cumin, and salt to the slow cooker.
2.Set for six hours on low.
3.At the end of six hours, stir in the chickpeas and zucchini.
4.Cook for another hour. Taste and adjust seasonings if needed.

Vegan Jambalaya

We all love Mardi Gras. With most of the festivities focusing on food, here is a delicious vegan jambalaya to make in the crockpot.

Servings: 4
Prep Time: 10 minutes
Ingredients:

- Pepper
- Himalayan Salt
- 6 oz. /168 g soy chorizo
- ¼ tsp /1 ¼ ml cayenne pepper
- 2 cups /480 ml cooked rice
- ½ tsp /2 ½ ml paprika
- 1 ½ cups /360 ml vegetable broth
- 1 chopped bell pepper
- ½ medium chopped onion
- 2 10 oz. cans /560 ml diced tomatoes with green chilies
- 1 cup /240 ml sliced okra
- 1 chopped celery stalk
- 2 cloves minced garlic

Instructions:
1. Add the chorizo to a skillet. Cook until browned and add to the crockpot.
2. Add the garlic, celery, onion, okra, and bell pepper to the crockpot.
3. Pour the tomatoes with their juices and broth over the top.
4. Add spices and stir. Set for six hours on low.
5. Add cooked rice. Give it a good stir. Serve and enjoy.

Indian Stew

This is similar to the traditional Indian recipe called Chana masala, which uses chickpeas. You could easily substitute chickpeas for the lentils. All of the vegetables pair beautifully together. It is a wonderful dish that makes your soul happy. It's gluten-free, vegetarian, and vegan-friendly. Spices have great anti-inflammatory properties and will help you boost your immune system!

Servings: 2
Ingredients:

- Pepper
- Salt
- 2 ½ cups /600 ml cooked lentils
- Juice of one lemon
- 1 tsp /5 ml garam masala
- 1 sweet potato, peeled and diced
- 2/3 cup /160 ml vegetable broth
- ½ tsp /2 ½ ml ground ginger
- 1 yellow bell pepper, chopped
- ¼ tsp /1 ¼ ml cayenne pepper
- 1 medium chopped onion
- 1 tbsp. /30 ml coriander
- 3 – 4 cloves minced garlic
- 1 15 oz. /420 g tomato sauce
- 1 tsp /5 ml turmeric
- 2 tsp /10 ml paprika
- 2 tsp /10 ml cumin

Instructions:
1. Add all ingredients to the slow cooker.
2. Set for three hours on high.
3. When sweet potatoes are tender, serve with brown rice.

<u>White Bean Soup</u>

Any white bean works well with this recipe. Cannellini, navy, or great northern will all make a flavorful and nutritious soup. You can keep this recipe simple by just using sun-dried tomatoes, onions, garlic, potatoes, carrots, and beans. It is a very versatile meal. You could also wilt in some greens after everything is cooked. You can even add corn or peas to add additional flavor. Get creative by adding in some vegan bacon or paprika for a smoky flavor. This is just a basic recipe. Go crazy and improvise! Use what you have on hand.

Servings: 10
Ingredients:

- Pepper
- 1 lb. /454 g dry white beans of choice, rinsed and sorted
- 1 – 2 tsp /5 – 10 ml dried dill
- 2 quarts /1.9 L vegetable broth
- Salt
- 1 medium chopped onion
- 1 pound /454 g frozen, sliced carrots
- 1 cup /240 ml chopped sun-dried tomatoes*
- 4 cloves garlic, smashed and peeled
- 3 – 4 tbsp. /45 – 60 ml fresh parsley, minced
- 2 medium potatoes, diced

Instructions:
1.Add the potatoes, beans, garlic, onion, broth, pepper, and salt to the slow cooker. Set for eight hours on low.
2.When beans are soft but not totally mushy, add dill, tomatoes, and carrots. Taste to see if you need any additional salt or pepper. Cook an additional 30 minutes.

*Look for dehydrated sun-dried tomatoes instead of the canned ones in oil. They are cheaper. Just rehydrate them in some water prior to putting them in the crockpot. You could add the liquid from the tomatoes to the soup for added flavor.

<u>Moroccan Coriander Soup</u>

If you are bored with your normal vegetable soup, try this flavorful Moroccan version to give your taste buds a boost.
Servings: 10
Prep Time: 15 minutes
Ingredients:

- Pepper
- Himalayan salt
- ¼ cup /60 ml olive oil
- 2 bunch fresh cilantro
- 3 medium chopped onions
- 8 cups /7.6 L low-sodium vegetable broth
- 1 head garlic
- 3 tbsp. /45 ml cumin
- 3 cinnamon sticks
- 3 tbsp. /45 ml coriander
- 4 14.5 oz. /870 g can chickpeas
- 2 bunches flat-leaf parsley
- 4 large chopped carrots
- 2 large peeled and chopped sweet potatoes
- 1 tsp /5 ml red pepper flakes
- 1 large peeled and chopped butternut squash
- 2 lb. /908 g red potatoes, chopped
- Toppings:
- 1 cup /240 ml chopped cilantro
- Agave
- 2 cups /480 ml cooked couscous

Instructions:
1.Tie the herbs together with some kitchen twine.
2.Add all ingredients except chickpeas and red potatoes to the crockpot. Set for eight hours on low.
3.At the six-hour mark, add the red potatoes.
4.Continue to cook an additional two hours.
5.Remove herbs and cinnamon sticks from the soup.
6.Stir in agave to sweeten.

7.Taste and adjust seasonings as needed. Serve the soup with couscous and chopped cilantro.

Tomato and Split Pea Soup

This is a hearty soup that warm you up on a chilly day. You can easily make it and freeze it in serving sizes so you always have a tasty meal on hand.

Servings: 4
Ingredients:

- Pepper
- Salt
- 6 sprigs fresh thyme
- 4 slices vegan bacon
- 1 large chopped onion
- 1 15 oz. /420 g can petite diced tomatoes
- 2 stalks chopped celery
- 2 tbsp. /10 ml Dijon mustard
- 2 medium chopped carrots
- 1 ½ cups /360 ml green split peas
- 4 cloves minced garlic
- Toppings:
- Chopped parsley
- Crisped vegan bacon

Instructions:
1.Cook vegan bacon in microwave until crisp.
2.Add 5 cups water, mustard, and tomatoes with juices.
3.Season with pepper and salt.
4.Add bacon, thyme, onion, celery, carrots, garlic, and split peas to slow cooker.
5.Cover. Set for 8 hours on low.
6.Take out thyme. Ladle into bowls.
7.Top with parsley and vegan bacon.

Butternut and White Bean Soup

This flavorful and hearty soup is filled with chickpeas, beans, and squash. It is great for warming you up on a cool fall evening.

Servings: 4
Prep Time: 20 minutes
Ingredients:

- Pepper
- Salt
- 1 15 oz. /420 g can chickpeas
- 1 tsp /5 ml coriander
- 1 15 oz. /420 g can cannellini beans
- 1 1-inch piece fresh ginger
- ¼ cup /60 ml fresh parsley
- 1 small chopped onion
- 1 chopped scallion
- 1 small peeled and chopped butternut squash
- ¼ cup /60 ml roasted pistachios
- 2 cloves minced garlic
- ½ cup /120 ml couscous
- 6 sprigs fresh thyme
- ¼ cup /60 ml dried apricots

Instructions:
1.In the slow cooker, stir together ½ tsp pepper, 1 tsp salt, 2 cups water, ginger, and coriander.
2.Add thyme, garlic, squash, and onion.
3.Cover. Set for five hours on low.
4.Twenty minutes before the soup is done, place couscous in bowl and pour 1 ¼ cups hot water over it.
5.Cover the bowl and allow it to set 15 minutes.
6.After time is up, fluff the couscous with a fork and add ¼ tsp pepper and salt, pistachios, scallion, and apricots.
7.In another bowl, mash half of the cannellini beans.
8.Turn cooker to high and stir in mashed beans.
9.Add in chickpeas and remaining cannellini beans.
10.Cook until hot. Ladle into bowls and top with couscous.

Red Thai Curry

This recipe is made simpler by making it in the crockpot. It's full of peas, mushrooms, cauliflower, and sweet potatoes. This is all smothered in a red coconut sauce. Using coconut milk will help you keep the fat content lower, but if you want full fat, by all means use the full-fat coconut milk.

Servings: 6 - 8
Prep Time: 15 minutes
Ingredients:

- Pepper
- Salt
- 1 cup /240 ml frozen or fresh green peas
- 1 -2 tsp /5 – 10 ml Sriracha sauce*
- 1 14 oz. /392 g can light coconut milk
- 2 medium sweet potatoes, cubed
- oz. /224 g quartered white mushrooms
- 1 small chopped onion
- 3 tbsp. /45 ml soy sauce
- ½ head cauliflower florets torn off
- 1 tbsp. /15 ml brown sugar
- 3 tbsp. /45 ml red curry paste*
- Cooked brown rice

Toppings:

- ½ cup /120 ml toasted cashews
- ¼ cup /60 ml chopped cilantro
- Fresh basil leaves

Instructions:
1.Place onion, sweet potatoes, and cauliflower in crockpot.
2.Combine Sriracha sauce, brown sugar, red curry paste, soy sauce, coconut milk, and salt.
3.Pour sauce over veggies. Stir to coat. Set at four hours on low. After four hours is over. Add mushrooms and peas. Cook an additional 30 minutes.
4.Serve with rice and top with toppings of choice.

Raw Food Soup Recipes

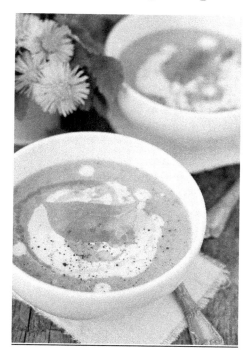

Watermelon Mint Soup

If saying something is sweet and cold and calling it soup is a little weird to you, you could call it a smoothie. This bowl of blended, fruity wonderfulness will have your taste buds doing a happy dance.

Servings: 4
Prep Time: 5 minutes

Ingredients:

- 2 tbsp. /30 ml mint leaves
- ¼ cup /60 ml coconut milk
- 1 tsp /5 ml baobab powder
- 1 tsp /5 ml acerola cherry powder
- 1 tbsp. /15 ml fresh ginger
- 3 cups /720 ml chopped watermelon, chilled
- 1 cup /240ml frozen strawberries
- ¾ cup /180 ml frozen cherries

Toppings:

- Watermelon cubes
- Frozen strawberries
- Frozen cherries
- Mint leaves

Instructions:
1.Put everything in your blender and mix until it is completely smooth.
2.Serve with toppings of your choice.

<u>Beetroot Soup</u>

This creamy chilled soup is great for when it is way too hot to turn on the stove. With its beautiful pink color, even the pickiest of eaters will enjoy this gazpacho.

Servings: 2
Prep Time: 5 minutes
Ingredients:

- Pepper
- Salt
- 1 tbsp. /15 ml lemon juice
- ½ ripe avocado pitted
- 1 small beetroot, peeled and chopped
- 1 tbsp. /15 ml chopped spring onion
- ½ small peeled cucumber
- 1 small chopped apple
- 1 cup /240 ml water
- 1 tbsp. /15 ml Shiro miso

Toppings:
- Fresh dill or herbs of your choice
- Favorite seeds

Instructions:
1.Add all ingredients except avocado to blender. Blend until smooth.
2.Add avocado and blend once more.
3.Taste and adjust seasonings if needed. Blend together.
Serve room temperature or chilled. Add toppings of your choice.

Curry Coconut Soup

This tasty soup can be served warm or chilled. Whichever way you decide, it is delicious. You will get warmed from the inside by the combination of spices in this easy recipe. It is sweet and savory with just the right amount of kick.

Servings: 2
Prep Time: 5 minutes
Ingredients:

- 2 tbsp. /30 ml chopped green onion
- 1 cup /240 ml shredded coconut
- 1 ½ cups /360 ml coconut water
- 2 tsp /10 ml curry powder
- 1 minced garlic clove
- 1 small chunked carrot
- ½ cup /120 ml water
- 2 cucumbers, julienned to make noodles
- 1 ½ tsp /7 ½ ml fresh ginger
- 1 handful cilantro
- 1 red bell pepper, cut into small sticks
- ½ Thai chili pepper, minced

Instructions:
1. Put the cilantro, cucumber noodles, and bell pepper sticks into a medium bowl.
2. Blend all other ingredients.
3. Blend 2 minutes to warm the soup.
4. If serving chilled, blend until creamy.
5. Pour over veggies.
6. Garnish with cilantro.

Ginger Watermelon Soup

Watermelon has always been a part of summer cookouts, and for a very good reason. Watermelon is very soothing to a body when it is hot. This refreshing soup combines the watermelon with tangy and cooling flavors to make a tantalizing flavor.

Servings: 4
Prep Time: 8 minutes
Ingredients:

- 5 cups /1.2 L watermelon
- 10 ice cubes
- ¼ cup /60 ml fresh lime juice
- ¾ tsp /3 ¾ ml salt
- 4 pitted Medjool dates
- 10 large mint leaves
- 2 tsp /10 ml fresh ginger

Instructions:
1.Add the ingredients to a blender. Blend for 20 seconds.
2.Pour into bowls.

Green Soup

Would you like to be able to make soup in ten minutes? This soup is a great way to get nourishment without standing over a hot stove. Blending the greens will ensure that their tough membranes get broken down so you can energize your body with each and every bite.

Servings: 2
Prep Time: 8 minutes
Ingredients:

- Pepper
- Salt
- 2 tbsp. /30 ml chopped onion
- 1 jalapeno, cored and seeded
- ½ cucumber, peeled
- 2 cups /470 ml spinach
- 1 lime, juiced
- 1 zucchini, chopped
- 2 celery stalks
- 1 avocado
- 1 to 1 ½ cups /240 to 360 ml water
- ¼ cup /60 ml parsley
- ¼ cup /60 ml cilantro

Instructions:
1.Add spinach and water to blender. Blend until smooth.
2.Add the rest of the ingredients one at a time until smooth and creamy.
3.You can serve immediately or chill for about an hour.
4.Garnish with chopped vegetables, hemp seeds, or dulse flakes.

<u>Almond Garlic Soup</u>

This is a great soup to give your immune system a boost if you are feeling under the weather. Creamy and light with lots of flavor. You will fall in love with this recipe.

Servings: 2
Prep Time: 5 minutes
Ingredients:
- Pepper
- Salt
- 1 tbsp. /15 ml olive oil
- ½ tsp /2 ½ ml apple cider vinegar
- 3 grated garlic cloves
- 1 ½ cups /360 ml cold almond milk
- Toppings:
- Olive oil
- Black pepper
- Lime wedges
- Fresh cilantro

Instructions:
1.Add everything to your blender and pulse until everything has become smooth.
2.Adjust seasonings as you see fit.
3.Serve with olive oil, black pepper, and lime juice. Store in refrigerator until ready to eat.

<u>Cantaloupe Soup</u>

Puree cantaloupe and orange juice to make a refreshing soup that can be eaten whenever you need to feel refreshed. It's great for breakfast as well.

Servings: 4
Prep Time: 10 minutes
Ingredients:

- 1/3 cup /80 ml orange juice
- 4 lime wedges
- 1 large cantaloupe, chilled

Instructions:
1.Put cantaloupe in blender.

2.Add orange juice.

3.Puree until smooth.

4.Pour into four bowls.

5.Squeeze over limes. Serve cold.

Tomato Gazpacho

A splash of hot sauce adds some zing to this classic gazpacho. This recipe is quick and easy because all you have to do is throw everything in the blender.

Servings: 6
Prep Time: 5 minutes
Ingredients:

- Pepper
- Salt
- 6 ice cubes
- 2 tbsp. /30 ml fresh lime juice
- 6 medium ripe tomatoes
- ½ cup /120 ml fresh cilantro leaves
- 2 medium English cucumbers
- Lime wedges
- 1 cup /240 ml corn kernels
- Hot sauce to taste

Instructions:
1.Put all ingredients in blender except lime wedges. Blend all ingredients until the mixture is the consistency you want.
2.If you are not going to serve this right away, place in an airtight container and refrigerate up to 24 hours.
3.Serve the soup with lime wedges and extra hot sauce.

<u>Spiced Fruit Soup</u>

When a soup is this colorful, you can add to the color by using white bowls. Let fresh seasonal fruit inspire you. For example, I use apricots in this recipe, but if peaches are in season, by all means, use them.

Servings: 5
Prep Time: 5 minutes
Ingredients:

- ¾ lb. /340.5 g apricots or other seasonal fruit
- A few drops of stevia
- 1 tbsp. /15 ml lemon zest
- 1 ½ pint /720 ml fresh raspberries
- 2 1-inch pieces of ginger
- 2 tbsp. /30 ml lemon juice
- 3 cups /720 ml water
- 2 whole star anise

Instructions:
1.Add 1 pint raspberries, lemon zest, star anise, ginger, water, and stevia to a pot.
2.Boil and mash the berries with a masher until they release their juices.
3.Use a mesh strainer to strain out seeds.
4.Put in large bowl.
5.Add lemon juice and apricot halves.
6.Chill for one hour in refrigerator.
7.Finish by add remaining raspberries into chilled broth. Ladle into bowls and serve.

Green Goddess Soup

If you have a goal to eat more greens daily, this soup is just the thing to do it. It is seasoned to perfection and super creamy. It has just enough lemon and shoyu to balance out the green flavor of the raw spinach. Tahini and avocado give you healthy fats and provide a creamy consistency. This pairs well with a kale salad.

Servings: 1
Prep Time: 5 minutes
Ingredients:

- 2 tbsp. /30 ml Nama shoyu
- 1 large handful spinach
- Juice of 1 lemon
- 1 date
- ½ peeled cucumber
- 1 medium cored bell pepper
- 1 tbsp. /30 ml raw tahini
- 1 small avocado

Instructions:
1.Add all ingredients to blender.
2.Add 1 ½ cups water and continue to blend.
3.Add more water to get desired consistency.
4.Enjoy now or chill for ten minutes.

<u>Spicy Gazpacho</u>

This is an oil and nut-free gazpacho. It has kick thanks to wonderful smoky chipotle powder. It's a great soup for that time between summer and fall when tomatoes bow out to sweet corn.

Servings: 2
Prep Time: 30 minutes
Ingredients:

- Himalayan salt
- 1 cup /240 ml corn kernels
- 1/3 cup /80 ml lime juice
- 1 cup /240 ml chopped zucchini
- 1 cup /240 ml chopped celery
- 1 small chopped onion
- 1 cup /240 ml sun-dried tomatoes, rehydrated with water
- 1 bunch cilantro
- 2 cups /470 ml chopped tomatoes
- Sliced avocado for garnish
- ½ tsp /2 ½ ml chipotle powder

Instructions:
1.Soak the sun-dried tomatoes in water for 20 minutes. Keep water.
2.Add all ingredients to blender. Blend well. Use water from tomatoes to make it blend more smoothly.
3.Pour half of the soup into bowl. Blend remaining soup in blender again to make it smoother. Pour into other soup. Stir in corn.
4.Serve the soup with the avocado.

Summer Vegetable Soup

This raw soup is inspired by all the summer gardens. If you love bell peppers, corn, basil, tomatoes, and zucchini, this soup is truly for you. Packed full of flavor, life, and vitality.

Servings: 4
Prep Time: 10 minutes
Ingredients:

- 1 tbsp. /15 ml miso
- 2 chopped bell peppers
- 2 tbsp. /30 ml nutritional yeast
- 2 cups /470 ml corn kernels
- 1 medium chopped zucchini
- ¼ cup /60 ml chopped basil
- 1 pitted date
- 1 tbsp. /15 ml apple cider vinegar
- 2 cups /470 ml quartered cherry tomatoes
- Salt
- 2 sun dried tomatoes
- 4 sliced scallions
- ¼ tsp /1 ¼ ml red pepper flakes
- 1 clove minced garlic
- 2 cups /470 ml water

Instructions:
1.Stir together scallions, basil, tomatoes, zucchini, peppers, and corn.
2.Take out 1/3 of mixture and put in blender with the remaining ingredients.
3.Blend until smooth.
4.Pour back over vegetables.
5.Let sit a couple hours in fridge.

Lemony Spinach Soup

Tangy and tart lemon brings out the flavors of baby spinach in this super easy soup. This soup is creamy and clean the perfect go-to for spring.

Servings: 2 - 3
Prep Time: 5 minutes
Ingredients:

- Pepper
- 4 cups /.95 L baby spinach
- 1 tbsp. /15 ml lemon zest
- 1 clove minced garlic
- 3 tbsp. /45 ml lemon juice
- 2 cups /470 ml nut milk
- 1 chopped scallion
- 3 tbsp. /45 ml white miso

Instructions:
1.Put all ingredients in blender. Blend until smooth.
2.You may garnish with avocado and black sesame seeds if you would like.

Epic Chili

If you love chili, I have a brand new raw chili for you to try. This recipe is absolutely raw, and nut and legume free. It also contains some sweet golden raisins. The blend of garlic, onion, cumin, salt, and chipotle gives this chili its flavor. While tomatoes, bell pepper, and mushrooms give it body. You may warm it a bit, but not too much. You could even add avocado to make it more filling.

Servings: 2
Prep Time: 8 minutes
Ingredients:

- Himalayan salt
- 2 tbsp. /30 ml diced red onion
- 1 large chopped Portobello cap
- 1 tsp /5 ml oregano
- ½ chopped red bell pepper
- 1 tbsp. /15 ml chili powder
- 1 tsp /5 ml cumin
- 2 large chopped tomatoes
- 1 – 2 dried chipotle pepper (adjust to your likeness)
- 1 handful golden raisins
- 1 clove minced garlic
- ¼ chopped onion
- 1 tsp /5 ml apple cider vinegar

Instructions:
1.Put red onion, bell pepper, and Portobello in bowl.
2.Place everything else in your blender and mix until it is all smooth
3.Pour over chopped vegetables.
4.Serve the soup with sliced avocado.

Sweet Corn and Tomato Soup

Blended soups are so quick and easy to make. This one is made with a base of tomatoes and sweet corn. Then it is blended into a creamy consistency with walnuts and hemp seeds. Seasoned with pepper, salt, dill, and garlic. It takes just minutes to make this soup. It's gluten-free, vegetarian, and vegan-friendly.

Servings: 1
Prep Time: 5 minutes
Ingredients:

- Pepper
- Salt
- Fresh or dried dill
- 1/3 cup sweet corn kernels
- ½ or whole chopped avocado
- 1 – 3 cloves minced garlic
- 1 chopped tomato
- 1 ½ cups /360 ml hot water
- Handful walnuts
- 1 – 2 tsp / 5 – 10 ml tamari
- Spoonful hemp seeds

Instructions:
1.Put water, tamari, hemp seeds, walnuts, garlic, corn, tomatoes, and half of the amount of avocado in a blender. Mix everything until combined and smooth.

2.Put in bowl. Stir in pepper and salt to suit your taste. Top with leftover avocado and dill.

Cucumber Pineapple Soup

This refreshing gazpacho is perfect for spring. It is full of spicy, sweet, bold flavors. The main thing there is to make sure the pineapple is very ripe. Just don't overdo it on the jalapeno. It's gluten-free, vegetarian, and vegan-friendly.

Servings: 4
Prep Time: 10 minutes
Ingredients:

- Salt
- 1 large English cucumber, chopped and peeled
- 1 cup /240 ml pineapple juice
- 1 large ripe pineapple, chopped, cored, and peeled
- Handful cilantro leaves, leave some for garnish
- ½ jalapeno, diced and seeded
- 1 tbsp. /15 ml lime juice
- 3 tbsp. /45 ml olive oil
- 1 chopped green onion

Instructions:

1.Place 3 cups pineapple and cucumber into food processor along with green onion, salt, lime juice, jalapeno, and pineapple juice. Pulse until smooth.

2.Add remaining cucumber, pineapple, ½ of the olive oil, and cilantro. Pulse a few times, but keep it chunky. Taste and adjust seasonings. Place in refrigerator to chill.

3.Serve with cilantro and a drizzle of olive oil.

<u>Avocado Apple Soup</u>

This is a beautiful soup that catches the eye and is great to give to guests. They will never know that they are eating a healthy soup.

Servings: 2
Prep Time: 5 minutes
Ingredients:
- Pepper
- 1 tbsp. /15 ml chopped onion
- Salt
- 1 chopped avocado
- 2 medium chopped apples
- 2 cups /480 ml water
- 2 tbsp. /30 ml olive oil
- Handful arugula leaves

Toppings:
- Minced onion
- Red pepper flakes

Instructions:
1.Leave some arugula for garnish.
2.Put water, olive oil, arugula leaves, chopped onion, apples, and avocado into a blender. Puree until smooth.
3.Add pepper and salt to taste. Place in bowls. Add arugula leaves, minced onion, and red pepper flakes.

Persimmon Pumpkin Soup

Juicy persimmon and pumpkin blend together perfectly with dates and almond milk, and you get to decide if it's a soup or a dessert. It's gluten-free, vegetarian, and vegan-friendly.

Servings: 2
Prep Time: 5 minutes
Ingredients:

- 3 – 5 dates
- ¾ cup /180 ml almond milk
- 2 – 3 persimmons with the top removed
- 1 cup /240 ml pumpkin pie puree
- Splash of vanilla
- Pinch of nutmeg

Instructions:
1.Add all ingredients to a blender. Blend until creamy.
2.Pour into a bowl or glass. You decide if it's a soup or smoothie.

Corn Chowder

This corn chowder is creamy and hearty. It is perfectly seasoned, and is very similar to traditional corn chowder, but healthier and more nourishing. You can use either a blender or food processor. It's gluten-free, vegetarian, and vegan-friendly.

Servings: 2
Prep Time: 5 minutes

Ingredients:
Creamy Chowder Base:

- Himalaya salt
- 1 cup /240 ml chopped zucchini
- 1 cup /240 ml macadamia nuts
- 1 tsp. /5 ml apple cider vinegar
- ½ cup /120 ml corn frozen or fresh
- ¼ cup /60 ml chopped mushrooms
- WATER:

Blender: 1 cup /240 ml water
Food processor: ½ to ¾ cup /120 – 180 ml water

Flavorings for the Chowder:

- 1 tbsp. /15 ml onion powder
- 1 tsp /5 ml dried parsley
- 1 tsp /5 ml ground celery seed
- Pepper to taste
- 1 tsp /5 ml kelp granules

Additional ingredients:

- ¼ cup /60 ml chopped carrot
- 1 cup /240 ml corn
- ¼ cup /60 ml chopped celery

Instructions:
1.Chowder Base: Add all base ingredients to blender and puree until creamy and whipped.Add in flavorings and pulse a couple of times to incorporate throughout.
2.To Assemble: Toss carrots, celery, and corn with pepper and salt. Mix all together and serve with dash of kelp granules.

Ginger Carrot Soup

Did you ever wonder how to make your carrot and ginger soup more appealing? How about blending in some orange juice and nut butter? Carrot and ginger are a great combination, but with the orange juice, it just gives the soup some extra kick that is just perfect for spring. You will be getting a bunch of beta carotene and vitamin C, plus a wonderful fresh flavor. It's gluten-free, vegetarian, and vegan-friendly.

Servings: 1
Prep Time: 5 minutes

Ingredients:

- 1-inch piece of ginger
- 1 tbsp. /15 ml nut butter of choice
- ½ cup /120 ml orange juice
- 2 large chopped carrots

Instructions:
1.Put all ingredients in blender. I usually start with the orange juice.
2.Blend until creamy.

Super Quick Recipes

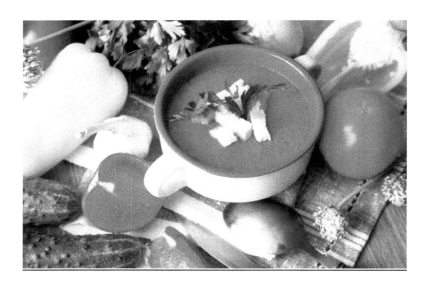

<u>Ginger Dumpling Soup</u>

This recipe is quick and easy. The hardest part is prepping all of the vegetables. These vegetables are quick-cooking, so once they are prepped, the cooking takes no time at all. The ginger in this recipe helps to fight inflammation like migraines, muscle soreness, and arthritis. It's vegetarian and vegan-friendly. To make this a gluten-free meal, look for gluten-free pot stickers in the freezer section.

Servings: 4
Prep Time: 20 minutes
Ingredients:

- Pepper
- Salt
- 1 tbsp. /15 ml rice vinegar
- 1 tbsp. /15 ml low-sodium soy sauce
- ½ head, small Napa cabbage, cut in bite-sized pieces
- 6 cups /1.44 L vegetable broth
- 1 1-inch piece ginger, sliced thin
- ½ small red chili, sliced thin
- 12 oz. frozen vegetable pot stickers
- 1 cup /240 ml snow peas, cut in half
- Sliced scallions

Instructions:
1.Put broth, ginger, and red chili in pot. Bring to boil. Add pot stickers and cabbage. Boil again for four minutes. Add peas. Simmer until vegetables are tender and pot stickers are cooked.
2.Add rice vinegar and soy sauce, stir.
3.Serve with sliced scallions.

Rice Noodle Soup

This is a fast soup to have any time you are craving something Asian. Rice noodles contain less fat than ramen, making them a healthy, yet tasty option. This soup is easily adaptable to any season. Change up the vegetables to what's fresh for the season. The only things you have to prep for the soup are your veggies and noodles. It's great garnished with chilies and some fresh lemon juice.

Servings: 6
Prep Time: 15 minutes
Ingredients:

- Lime wedge
- 2 tsp /10 ml salt
- Jalapeno, sliced
- Seasonal vegetables
- 1 tbsp. /30 ml vegetable oil
- Fried tofu cubes, optional
- ¼ c /60 ml red bell pepper, sliced
- 2 garlic cloves, chopped
- ¼ c /60 ml cremini mushrooms, sliced
- ¼ tsp /1.25 ml pepper
- 1 small onion, chopped
- oz. /196 g dried vermicelli rice noodles

Instructions:
1. Begin by prepping the noodles. Put the noodles in six cups of boiling water. Allow to sit, covered, for two minutes. Drain them and rinse in cold water.
2. Begin frying the onion in a pan until they have become golden, about two minutes. Stir in garlic and allow the mixture to cook for 30 minutes. Pour in six cups of boiling water, add pepper and salt.
3. As the broth simmers, chop up the herbs, pepper, and mushrooms.
4. Mix in the herbs, pepper, mushrooms, and any other seasonal vegetables that you want to the broth. Allow this to simmer for a couple of minutes, or until you like the tenderness of the vegetables.
5. Take off of the heat Place some rice noodles in a bowl and ladle on some of the broth. Top with lime wedge and jalapeno.

<u>Coconut Curry</u>

This is a vegan and gluten-free 30-minute meal. It is packed full of veggies that are swimming in a deliciously coconut milk broth. To top it all off, it is topped with a coconut quinoa. It's so delicious that you won't believe it's good for you.

Servings: 4
Prep Time: 5 minutes

Ingredients:
Curry:

- Pepper
- Salt
- 1 cup /240 ml veggie stock
- 2 14-oz /396 g cans coconut milk
- Pinch cayenne (optional)
- 1 tbsp. /8 g curry powder
- 1/3 cup /28 g snow peas
- 1 tbsp. /15 ml coconut oil
- ¼ cup /45 g diced tomatoes
- ½ cup /64 g diced carrots
- ½ cup /45 g broccoli florets
- 1 tbsp. /6 g grated ginger
- 4 cloves minced garlic
- 1 small onion, diced

Quinoa:

- 1 cup /170 g quinoa, rinsed
- 1 14-oz /396 g can coconut milk
- 1 tbsp. /15 ml agave

Instructions:
1.Start by prepping the quinoa by rinsing it in a mesh strainer. Toast the quinoa for about three minutes. Pour in a can of coconut milk and a half cup of water. Allow to boil, and then reduce to a simmer. Cover pot and let cook 15 minutes. Liquid should be absorbed.

2.While the quinoa is cooking, heat oil and sauté the broccoli, carrot, ginger, garlic, and onion. Season to your liking with pepper and salt.

3.Stir frequently until the veggies have softened, around five minutes.

4.Mix in another pinch of salt, coconut milk, veggie stock, cayenne, and curry powder. Let the mixture simmer for about ten to 15 minutes.

5.Stir in the tomatoes and snow peas during the last five minutes.

6.Adjust the taste as needed, adding more pepper or salt.

7.Serve the curry over a helping of the coconut quinoa. Garnish with any herbs that you would like, and squeeze on some fresh lemon juice.

Plant Based Pho

Another delicious 30-minute Asian inspired dish, but this pho doesn't take three hours to cook. This is a quick pho that you can make as any weeknight meal. This is a crowd pleaser and easy to adjust in any way that you want. The fun part is getting to fix your bowl yourself.

Servings: 4 to 6
Prep Time: 10 minutes
Ingredients:

- 8-oz /224 g bean sprouts
- 14-oz /392 g rice noodles, cooked
- 2 tsp /10 ml sesame oil
- 2 jalapeno peppers, sliced
- 6 oz. /168 g shiitake mushrooms stems removed
- 6 green onions, sliced
- 1 ½ tbsp. /22.5 ml vegan butter
- Salt
- 1 ½ tbsp. /22.5 ml hoisin sauce
- 1 tbsp. /15 ml grated ginger
- 64 oz. /1796 g vegetable broth

Instructions:
1.Mix the salt, ginger, onion, and broth in a large pot. Allow to come to a rolling boil. Turn down the heat and allow to simmer for 15 minutes.
2.As the broth cooks, warm the butter in a skillet. Sauté the mushrooms for around six minutes. Mix in the sesame oil and hoisin sauce. Cook until everything has thickened and the mushrooms are coated. Take it off the heat.
3.Place the cooked noodles in four to six bowls. Fill each of the bowls with some of the broth. Top with cilantro, basil, mushrooms, jalapenos, and bean sprouts. Serve the pho with chili garlic sauce, hoisin, and a lime wedge.

Moroccan Carrot Soup

This is a simple carrot soup with lots of spices. Add some crunch with the toasted pumpkin seeds.

Servings: 6
Prep Time: 15 minutes
Ingredients:

- ½ tsp /2 ½ ml coriander
- Pepper
- ½ tsp /2 ½ ml cinnamon
- Salt
- 6 tbsp. /180 ml olive oil
- ¼ tsp /1 ¼ ml cayenne pepper
- 5 cups /1.2 L vegetable broth
- 1 tsp /5 ml cumin
- 3 cups /720 ml cooked carrots
- ½ cup /120 ml toasted pumpkin seeds
- ¼ tsp /1 ¼ ml allspice

Instructions:
1.Add the carrots and broth to blender. Puree until smooth.
2.Put mixture in a pot. Add in salt and spices. Cook about 8 minutes.
3.Add water until it is at the desired consistency.
4.Serve soup with pumpkin seeds, ground pepper, and drizzle with olive oil.

Loaded Veggie Soup

If you have ever doubted that vegetables can taste good, you have to try this filling soup. Loaded with cannellini beans and a ton of veggies and flavored with Italian seasoning.

Servings: 8
Prep Time: 5 minutes
Ingredients:

- Pepper
- Himalayan salt
- 3 15 oz./420 g cannellini beans
- 1 cup /240 ml frozen peas
- 1 15 oz. /420 g diced tomatoes
- oz. /224 g broccoli rabe, remove thick stems
- 1 large chopped onion
- 1 medium chopped zucchini
- 6 garlic cloves, minced
- ½ small butternut squash
- 2 tsp /10 ml Italian seasoning
- 1 fennel bulb or 4 celery stalks

Instructions:

1.Work in batches if you need to. Puree beans and tomatoes with juices. Pour into pot.

2.Add 4 cups water, pepper and salt to taste, Italian seasoning, garlic, and onion. Bring to a boil and allow it to cook for ten minutes.

3.Place in broccoli rabe, zucchini, squash, and fennel. Simmer vegetables until soft, around 20 minutes. Mix in peas and let them heat through.

4.Serve drizzled with oil.

<u>Creamy Vegetable Soup</u>

This recipe is simple to make. It is healthy and comforting. Just throw a bunch of vegetables into a pot with herbs and stock and simmer. Finish it off with some coconut milk.

Servings: 4
Prep Time: 5 minutes
Ingredients:

- Pepper
- Salt
- 1 tbsp. /15 ml olive oil
- ¼ cup /60 ml coconut milk
- 3 sprigs fresh thyme
- 3 medium red potatoes, chunked
- 4 celery stalks, cut into ½-inch pieces
- 3 garlic cloves, halved
- 3 cups /720 ml vegetable stock
- 1 lb.454 g carrots, peeled cut into ½-inch pieces
- ¼ tsp /1 ¼ ml red pepper flakes
- 1 large chopped onion
- 2 bay leaves

Instructions:

1.Heat oil in pan. Add celery, carrots, and onions. Add ½ tsp. salt and red pepper flakes. Cook until soft.

2.Add potatoes, thyme, bay leaves, and garlic. Cook about 5 minutes.

3.You may add oil if the pan gets too dry.

4.Add stock and boil. Simmer until potatoes are fork tender.

5.Take soup off heat. Remove thyme sprigs and bay leaves and discard. Use an immersion blender and mix until you get a smooth consistency.

6.Mix in the coconut milk. Adjust seasoning if needed.

<u>Chickpea Vegetable Soup</u>

A comforting vegetable soup that's packed full of chickpeas and tons of veggies. It is so easy to make. Just put everything in a pot and simmer

Servings: 6
Prep Time: 10 minutes
Ingredients:

- Pepper
- Salt
- 1 tbsp. /15 ml vegan margarine
- 3 cups /720 ml low-sodium vegetable broth
- 1 medium chopped onion
- ½ tsp /2 ½ ml turmeric
- 4 minced garlic cloves
- 1 cup /240 ml water
- 3 carrots, sliced into rounds
- 1 14.5 oz. /406 g diced tomatoes
- 4 celery stalks, sliced thin
- 2 tbsp. /30 ml olive oil
- 2 15 oz. /420 g cans chickpeas, drained and rinsed
- 1 bay leaf

Instructions:
1.Heat oil and margarine in a pot.
2.Add bay leaf, garlic, celery, carrots, onions, pepper, and salt. Cook until veggies are tender.
3.Add tomatoes, chickpeas, and turmeric.
4.Add water and broth. Stir to combine. Bring to boil.
5.Allow it to simmer for ten minutes. Take off heat.
6.Taste and adjust seasonings if needed.
7.Serve, garnished with parsley.

Peanut and Sweet Potato Soup

This soup's savory exotic mix of flavors will spice up any meal.

Servings: 4
Prep Time: 20 minutes
Ingredients:

- Pepper
- Himalayan salt
- Roasted peanuts, chopped
- Cilantro
- ½ cup /120 ml creamy peanut butter
- 2 tbsp. /30 ml olive oil
- 4 garlic cloves, minced
- 1 15 oz. /420 g diced tomatoes
- 2 tsp /10 ml cumin
- 1 large chopped onion
- 1 ½ lb. /680 g sweet potatoes, peeled and chopped
- ¼ tsp /1 ¼ ml cayenne
- 2 tbsp. /30 ml fresh grated ginger

Instructions:
1.Heat oil in a pan. Add onion, season with pepper and salt. Cover and cook until tender.
2.Add ginger and garlic. Stir. Add cayenne and cumin. Stir. Add sweet potatoes and stir to combine.
3.Add water, peanut butter, and tomatoes. Allow the water to boil. Cover and allow to cook until sweet potatoes can easily be pierced
4.with a fork.
5.Serve the soup with peanuts and cilantro.

Breakfast Miso Soup

A satisfying, quick soup that you will be able to eat in 30 minutes or less. This soup is packed with lots of nutrition for a savory and warm start to your day. It's delicious for breakfast or anytime you are hungry.

Servings: 4
Prep Time: 10 minutes
Ingredients:

- Pepper
- Salt
- 2 tbsp. /30 ml olive oil
- ½ chopped onion
- 2 minced garlic cloves
- 2 tbsp. /30 ml white miso
- 1 cup /240 ml broccoli florets
- 2 diced celery stalks
- 1 cup /240 ml cooked chickpeas
- 2 peeled and diced carrots

Instructions:
1. Heat oil in pan. Add onion, carrots, celery, and garlic. Let sauté until the veggies become tender.
2. Mix in chickpeas and broccoli. Cook for two minutes.
3. Add four cups water. Allow to come to a boil. Cook until veggies are tender.
4. Take off heat.
5. Add in the miso and stir until dissolved.
6. Taste and add pepper and salt as needed.

15-Minute White Bean Soup

This is a perfect recipe for those of us who hates spending all day in the kitchen. This fiber-rich soup uses canned beans and stock for an easy and quick meal for evenings when you don't feel like cooking.

Servings: 2
Prep Time: 5 minutes
Ingredients:

- 1 ½ tsp /7 ml lemon juice
- Pepper
- Himalayan salt
- 1 clove minced garlic
- 2 tsp /10 ml olive oil
- 2 thinly sliced scallions
- 1 15 oz. /420 g can white beans, rinsed and drained
- ½ tsp / 2 ½ ml oregano

Instructions:
1. Heat oil in pan. Add oregano, garlic, and scallions. Sauté until soft.
2. Add beans and broth. Stir. Cook until hot.
3. Mash beans with spoon or potato masher to help thicken soup.
4. Add lemon juice. Stir well. Season with pepper and salt.

Coconut and Corn Soup

This combination of coconut milk and sweet corn creates a soup that tastes surprising, familiar, and fresh from the farm.

Servings: 4
Prep Time: 5 minutes
Ingredients:

- Pepper
- Himalayan salt
- 1 tbsp. /15 ml fresh lime juice
- 2 ½ cups /600 ml water
- 3 cups /720 ml fresh corn kernels
- 1 jalapeno chili, seeded and chopped
- 1 14 oz. can /392 g light coconut milk

Instructions:

1.Add water, coconut milk, corn kernels, and jalapeno to pot. Bring to boil. Simmer until corn is tender.

2.Use immersion blender to puree soup. Strain through sieve and discard solids. Season mixture to your taste.

3.Allow it to chill for three hours or overnight. Add lime juice. Stir.

4.Garnish with fresh corn and sprinkle each serving with pepper.

Thai Tofu Soup

This Asian recipe is quick and easy. Be careful with the red curry paste. It can get rather warm. If you like it hot, by all means, add more. If you like it milder, reduce the amount. Check the curry paste's ingredients. Sometimes they are manufactured with non-vegetarian ingredients.

Servings: 4
Prep Time: 15 minutes
Ingredients:

- Himalayan salt
- 1 tsp /5 ml Thai red curry paste
- 1 tsp /5 ml grated fresh ginger
- 2 cups /470 ml low-sodium vegetable broth
- 4 oz. /112 g snow peas
- ¼ cup /60 ml torn basil leaves
- 1 14 oz. can /392 g coconut milk
- 14 oz. /392 g extra-firm tofu, drained and cubed
- 2 tbsp. /30 ml fresh lime juice
- ½ lb. /227 g mushrooms, sliced thin
- 2 carrots, halved lengthwise, sliced into half moons
- 4 oz. /112 g green beans, halved
- Asian chili garlic sauce

Instructions:
1.Mix the curry paste and ginger together in a pot. Pour in the broth and coconut milk along with a teaspoon of salt. Whisk until smooth and bring to a boil.
2.Add mushrooms, carrots, and green beans. Simmer until tender.
3.Add tofu and snow peas until peas turn bright green.
4.Stir in lime juice. Sprinkle on basil and chili garlic sauce.

Summer Minestrone Soup

This recipe is a lighter version of traditional minestrone soup. It's great to boost your immune system and beat inflammation, which we know is the cause behind most diseases.

Servings: 4
Prep Time: 10 minutes
Ingredients:

- Pepper
- Himalayan salt
- 2 cloves minced garlic
- 1 cup /240 ml fresh corn kernels
- ½ cup /120 ml frozen peas
- 4 cups /.95 L low-sodium vegetable broth
- 1 large chopped onion
- 1 small chopped carrot
- ½ bunch basil
- 1 tbsp. /15 ml olive oil
- 1 small chopped yellow squash
- 1 small chopped zucchini
- oz. /224 g red potatoes

Instructions:
1.Heat oil in a pan. Add onion and sprinkle with pepper and salt.
2.Cover and simmer until onions turn translucent. Uncover and allow to cook until the onions have become tender and browned slightly.
3.Chop 1 tablespoon basil stems and add to onions and garlic. Add broth and potatoes. Simmer 5 minutes.
4.Add carrot, squash, and zucchini. Simmer 3 minutes. Add corn and peas. Continue to cook until veggies are tender.
5.Serve the soup with a sprinkle of basil.

<u>White Bean and Kale Soup</u>

Fresh vegetables like butternut squash and kale along with beans that are high in fiber make this soup loaded with lots of health-boosting nutrients.

Servings: 4
Prep Time: 15 minutes
Ingredients:

- Pepper
- Salt
- 2 tbsp. /30 ml olive oil
- 2 stalks chopped celery
- 1 large chopped onion
- 1 15 oz. /420 g can low-sodium white beans
- 1 medium chopped butternut squash
- 2 tbsp. /30 ml tomato paste
- 2 cloves minced garlic
- 1 bunch kale
- cups /7.6 L vegetable broth
- 16 sprigs fresh thyme

Instructions:

1.Heat oil in a pot. Add onion. Sprinkle with pepper and salt. Cover and simmer until onion becomes soft. Stir thyme, garlic, and celery.

2.Let them cook until onion is slightly browned. Add tomato paste and continue to cook.

3.Add broth and squash. Simmer until the squash becomes tender. Mix in kale and beans. Let it cook until kale is tender. Discard thyme sprigs before serving.

Quinoa Chickpea Soup

Quinoa is fast cooking and adds a nutty flavor to this healthy, delicious soup. Quinoa is an excellent protein source for vegetarians and vegans.

Servings: 4
Prep Time: 15 minutes
Ingredients:
- Pepper
- Himalaya salt
- ½ cup /120 ml quinoa
- 1 stalk chopped celery
- 2 tbsp. /30 ml red wine vinegar
- 2 cups /470 ml low-sodium vegetable broth
- 1 medium chopped onion
- 1 tbsp. /15 ml paprika
- 2 15 oz. cans /840 g chickpeas
- 1 medium chopped carrot
- 1 chopped red bell pepper
- 2 tbsp. /30 ml olive oil
- 3 cloves minced garlic
- 1 chopped yellow bell pepper
- Chopped fresh parsley

Instructions:
1.Cook quinoa according to directions on package.
2.Heat oil in Dutch oven. Add celery, carrot, and onion. Cover. Cook until soft.
3.Add pepper, salt, paprika, and garlic. Add bell peppers and continue to cook.
4.Add 1 cup water, broth, and chickpeas. Cook until the vegetables are tender. Mix in vinegar and quinoa.
5.Serve the soup with chopped parsley.

Vegan Sausage and Kale Soup

This soup goes from stove to table in under 35 minutes. It is loaded with heart-healthy kale, vegan sausage, potatoes, garlic, and onion in vegetable broth.

Servings: 6
Prep Time: 10 minutes
Ingredients:

- oz. /224 g vegan sausage
- 1 tbsp. /15 ml minced garlic
- 3 medium chopped Yukon Gold potatoes
- 1 medium chopped onion
- 12 oz. /336 g kale, tough stems removed and chopped
- 6 cups /1.44 L low-sodium vegetable broth
- Red pepper flakes to garnish

Instructions:
1.Heat Dutch oven. Cook the sausage until it is browned.

2.Add garlic and onion. Continue to cook until onion softens. Add broth and bring to a boil.

3.Add kale and potatoes. Simmer. Cover partially. Cook until potatoes are tender.

4.Serve the soup with red pepper flakes.

Potato Leek Soup

Potato soup is usually full of ingredients that are very fatty, and typically contains lots of cream. This vegetable broth version is healthier and lighter, but still very comforting.

Servings: 4
Prep Time: 15 minutes
Ingredients:
- Pepper
- Salt
- 2 tbsp. /30 ml olive oil
- 2 medium chopped leeks
- 1 cup /240 ml frozen peas
- 2 stalks chopped celery
- 1 tbsp. /15 ml fresh lemon juice
- cups /7.6 L low-sodium vegetable broth
- 1 medium chopped fennel bulb
- 1 ½ lbs. /681 g red potatoes
- 4 cloves minced garlic
- 6 large fresh dill sprigs

Instructions:
1.Heat oil in a pot. Add fennel, celery, and leeks. Sprinkle with pepper and salt. Cook just until vegetables are soft. Add garlic and continue to cook.
2.Tie dill sprigs together. Add to the pot with broth and potatoes. Bring to a boil, then reduce to a simmer. Cook until potatoes can easily be pierced by a fork.
3.Add celery and peas and heat through. Discard dill sprigs. Add lemon juice and stir. Add more chopped dill if desired.

Creamy Cauliflower Soup

This dreamy soup is effortless. Not much dicing or chopping. Just break off the florets and chop up the stalk with potatoes, onions, and some garlic. Throw them in a pot with some broth and coconut milk. When tender, give it a whirl with an immersion blender, and there you have it. This recipe works well with any vegetable that gets tender when boiled. Vegetables like zucchini, fennel, peas, beetroot, potatoes, parsnips, carrots, or broccoli work perfectly.

Servings: 4
Prep Time: 10 minutes
Ingredients:

- Pepper
- Salt
- 2 cloves chopped garlic
- 2 cups/470 ml coconut milk
- 2 lb. /908 g cauliflower (1 medium head), florets taken off and stalk chopped roughly
- 1 large chopped onion
- 2 cups /470 ml vegetable stock
- oz. /250 g potatoes (1 large, 2 small), peeled and chopped

Toppings:

- Thyme
- Coconut milk, to drizzle
- Olive oil, to drizzle

Instructions:
1.Add all ingredients except pepper and salt to pot. Bring to boil.
2.Simmer until cauliflower is soft.
3.Using an immersion blender, mix until everything is smooth. Stir in some pepper and salt to your liking.
4.If soup appears too thick, add more milk or broth. If you want the soup thicker, let it boil for a bit longer.
5.Serve the soup with thyme. Drizzle with olive oil and milk.

Classic Vegetable Soup

This is a delicious recipe and very easy to throw together. Just some chopping and then let it simmer until you have to soup that's a keeper. This is one your family will ask for over and over again. It uses some fresh as well as frozen vegetables, so you get the freshness but also the ease of using frozen. It's gluten-free, vegetarian, and vegan-friendly.

Servings: 7
Prep Time: 15 minutes
Ingredients:

- Pepper
- Salt
- 1 cup /240 ml fresh or frozen peas
- 1 medium chopped onion
- 1 1/4 cups /300 ml corn
- 4 medium chopped carrots
- 4 14.5 oz. cans /1624 g low-sodium vegetable broth
- 2 ½ tbsp. /32 ½ ml olive oil
- 1 ½ cups /360 ml fresh or frozen green beans
- 3 stalks chopped celery
- 2 14.5 oz. cans /812 g diced tomatoes
- ½ tsp /2.5 ml dried thyme
- 1 cloves minced garlic
- 2 bay leaves
- 1/3 cup /80 ml fresh chopped parsley
- 3 medium peeled and chopped potatoes

Instructions:

1. Heat oil in a Dutch oven. Add celery, carrots, and onions. Cook a few minutes and add garlic.
2. Add broth, thyme, bay leaves, parsley, potatoes, and tomatoes.
3. Season with pepper and salt. Bring to a boil and add green beans.
4. Simmer until potatoes are tender. Add peas and corn and cook an additional five minutes.
5. Serve warm.

More books by Elena Garcia available at:

www.YourWellnessBooks.com

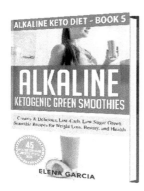

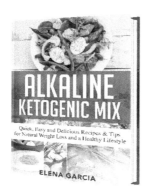

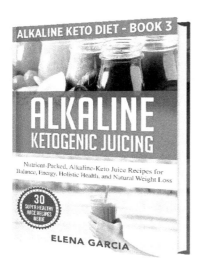

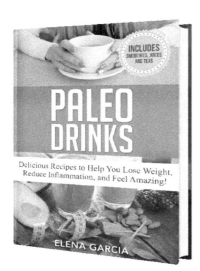

CPSIA information can be obtained
at www.ICGtesting.com
Printed in the USA
BVHW042356270720
584757BV00009B/196